Rebirthing in the New Age

To Hal Kramer, the publisher,
for having the guts to publish this book.
It just might change history.

We want to acknowledge the true source
of everything good and right and loving,
God the Almighty, the "Presence."

Rebirthing in the New Age

Leonard Orr
and
Sondra Ray

Celestial Arts
Berkeley, California

The authors are grateful to the following people who contributed
portions of this book:

Elana Lynse	Bobby Birdsall
Rick Fields	Phil Du Bois, M.D.
Gary Sohler	Fred Lehrman
Kristian Kelly	Bill Chapelle

First Printing, November 1977
Cover drawing by Colleen Forbes
Revised edition: first printing, May 1983
Made in the United States of America

Library of Congress Cataloging in Publication Data

Orr, Leonard.
    Rebirth for a new age.

    1. Self-actualization (Psychology) 2. Consciousness.
3. Childbirth—Psychological aspects. I. Ray, Sondra,
joint author. II. Title.
BF637.S4077   158   76-53337
ISBN 0-89087-134-5

    10   11   12   13   14   -   87   86   85

Contents

Should new age wine come in old age bottles?

The authors of this book do not presume to be writers in the traditional sense. We have spared ourselves the effort of trying to force our intuition and experience into the mold of an "objective" scientific presentation. What follows is simply what we have observed to be true stated in the language with which we communicate among ourselves. We feel that this will best convey the energy of the process which we have undergone together in the Rebirthing Community. We hope that more books will follow as a result of this one, and we invite members of the scientific fraternity to join us in exploring this work.

As self-established, homegrown, grassroots American gurus, we allow ourselves the pleasure of speaking our minds among friends. We are happy to be making your acquaintance.

Fred Lehrman

A letter from the author to you. . .

There are a few things that I would like to let you know about this book:

- You will never regret having read it; it may change your perceptions but you won't be sorry.

- Rebirthing has changed dramatically since this book was written. It has become easier, less traumatic, more pleasurable, and much faster. I feel that it is important to leave this book as it is because it reveals what it was like in the beginning.

- Please do not let anything that I had to go through frighten you. I was willing to become a human guinea pig to help develop the knowledge and understanding which we now possess. You will benefit directly from this early research and discover that Rebirthing can be delightful.

- It is the best gift that you could ever give yourself. You deserve it.

- This book is my personal gift to you and will make your rebirths easier.

Love,

Sondra Ray!

A Tribute to Rebirthing and California

I love this book, and yet for years I have been trying to Rebirth it! However, every time I attempted to rewrite it, redo it, update it, change it or revise it, the manuscripts would be lost or mysteriously "dematerialized." Even the copies of the changes were lost by the publishing house, which almost never happens. I finally accepted the fact that, for some reason, this book is supposed to be left exactly the same as we wrote it, embarrassing as some sections are to me, for historical purposes, and especially for the training of Rebirthers and anyone else. It was part of my training and it worked. I can still recommend this book highly. It is educational, and the information in it has been always incredibly valuable to me. I use it daily in my own life and it works. However, Rebirthing has changed, matured, been perfected and smoothed out in the last seven years. My new book *Celebration of Breath* moves Rebirthing to the level it is today. Since we are only in the first decade of Rebirthing, I am sure it will continue to evolve to higher and higher levels. I have noticed that Rebirthers love it more every year.

When I wrote this book I was a "babe in the metaphysical woods." I wanted answers and results in my life. I became totally willing to be a complete student and devotee of the process and Leonard. I allowed Leonard to be my complete teacher. He became my mother, my father, my obstetrician and my guru. I became as helpless and as ridiculous as I needed to be to knock off my ego. At times I was like an infant and could not think for myself. Whatever I did, as embarrassing as it is, it worked for me. I am what I am today as a result. I do not mean to imply, however, that everyone has to go through what we went through as pioneers. First of all, we started Rebirthing backwards. In the beginning it was very dramatic and hard because of this. We have now mastered it, so that new people coming to Rebirthing do not necessarily have to go through what we did. We no longer start out people with wet Rebirthing, for example. This turned out to be "too much, too fast." So, again, I want to make it very plain that your rebirth experiences do not in any way need to be like mine were in the beginning. We were pioneers, and we did not know what we were doing when we began this. It was all experimental.

Some people may be "turned off" by what could look like the "California hype" type of "movement" I talk about in the beginning. I could take that part out and just leave you with all the incredible "data." You could also skip that part and study the other information. However, I find that reading what it was like to be a pioneer of this work gives it more flavor and helps one to really appreciate it. Besides, I personally want to acknowledge the State of California and the City of San Francisco for providing the "space" for me to be as outrageous as I am outrageous in my research. I always felt people in California were cheering us on while we were spending two years down in a basement in a tub of water at approximately 106° (which was too hot). The fact that I worked all day and all night in the nude did not make a difference to me or anyone. We never even worried about it. We were too thrilled with the results of this work to be concerned with that.

It was rather hard "delivering" Rebirthing to the world because, for one thing, it came out "breech." We had it all backwards at first, and many times it was almost more than we could handle at a given time. So, in a way, we as Rebirthers are still trying to heal Rebirthing of its own birth trauma. I have, as always, a very high intention to "Rebirth Rebirthing" and deliver it just right to the world. I have prayed a lot that the media would co-operate with the sacredness of it and give it the high respect that it deserves. I still feel hurt when someone puts it down as a California hype. I want it to be very clear that Rebirthing to me is very sacred. I see it as a rite of passage spiritually, and I will always acknowledge California where Rebirthing "grew up" and was nurtured its first years of life. We are now taking Rebirthing to all other states and many foreign countries. Leonard is presently residing at Campbell Hot Springs (which is especially good as a wet Rebirthing training cetner) near Lake Tahoe, California.

Our research in Life Extension and the philosophy of Physical Immortality continues deeply. I feel that I am only beginning to integrate Chapter 5 of this book with *A Course In Miracles* and the teachings of Babaji, the Yogi Christ of India. Although that chapter is obviously not the last word on this subject, I am still quite convinced that it is important to master the Immortality principles before one can become a true spiritual master and ulti-mately dematerialize and rematerialize at will. One of my favorite books *The Door of Everying* (especially Chapter 11) has really assisted me to bring all this together in my mind. Every year my understanding of this information becomes clearer and Babaji teaches me as fast as I can learn. I feel very humbled by the mys-tical experiences I have had in rebirthing and meditation that have convinced me even physiologically of the truth of these teachings. When I am able to write about these without ego involvement, I will.

I suggest you take your time digesting this book. Please remem-ber to breathe fully while taking it in. I invite you to read my other books; and I must say that I feel every book I write is better than the one before because I am clearer and more free and enlightened with more joy and love. It may be best to study the books in the order that I wrote them, since to every book I bring more and more energy and a book builds on the ones before.

1. *I Deserve Love* (affirmations on love, sex and relationships)
2. *Rebirthing in the New Age* (the birth and development of Re-birthing)

3. *Loving Relationships* (how your birth and family patterns affect relationships)
4. *The Only Diet There Is* (spiritual diets for mastering the body)
5. *Celebration of Breath* (Rebirthing today—Part II)
6. *The Ideal Birth* (preparation, especially before conception, for
   bringing a new being into the world and latest developments in
   birthing, such as underwater birth)

I sincerely feel that my writing career is just beginning and I in-
tend always to be writing a book. It is also my intention to be in an
eternal relationship with you, the reader of my books, and I do experience loving you and appreciating your willingness to apply
these teachings to your life so that we can improve the quality of
life forever.

A letter from Leonard to you...

The main dilemma in writing a book about spiritual matters is that the harder we tried to say it right the more difficult it became. It occurred to us that if we tried to make it perfect this book would never get published. This is true about talking in seminars, too. A basic spiritual concept is that not only does our interpretation of the facts change, but the facts themselves also can change and be transformed.

This book is about real human lives being transformed by spiritual truth. The individuals reported on here at present bear little or no resemblance to themselves as they were during the report. Plus, a report by Sondra or Leonard can at best be only a partial picture of a real divine human being. As is illustrated by our presentations of each other, we change so fast our perceptions or conclusions of each other are more accurately described as projections or reflections.

It is best to practice full disclosure of oneself and be comfortable about the potential embarrassment. We have found that telling the truth about ourselves is the best way to permanent bliss and success in the real world.

Therefore you may find that this book is more about the experience of *your* spiritual evolution than ours. People who are around us much say that they experience their highest highs and lowest lows but if they practice the truths we represent we have noticed that they accumulate more success and bliss with every cycle. We see hundreds of people who have "hung out" with us for a few years whose lives are filled with peace, love, health, and all kinds of worldly success. There are spots in this book that we would change, delete, or apologize for if we were to work on it more. We could work on it and improve it forever. However, I think it is more intelligent to trust you, the reader, to edit it for your own personal growth. Feel free to throw out, change, or skip whatever shocks you or goes over your head. Stick with the parts that feed your soul personally. Reread the parts that stimulate movement in your mind, love in your heart, and self-esteem in your spirit. You may also find parts that you will have to balance with your own interpretations of reality.

It is our wish that this book will be an enlightening, pleasurable, and practical experience for you.

It is impossible to tell when I conceived of Theta seminars, since it is the product of my whole life, but it became a legal form in August 1974. Rebirth International was founded in 1976. Prosperity International was founded in 1977.

L.O.

Warning:

"This Book May Be Hazardous to Your Misery."

—Bobby Birdsall

Preface to the Revised edition

The rebirthing movement has gone a long way since *Rebirthing in the New Age* was published in 1977. Then there were only a few thousand people practicing conscious connected breathing rhythm; now there are over a million people doing it, and the students of breath multiply rapidly. The reason it is spreading so rapidly is that conscious breathing is usually more pleasurable than eating when done on a daily basis, and the first ten or even hundreds of energy cycles can produce full body orgasmic feeling that can be enjoyed for a full hour or more.

Rebirthing can be more pleasurable than food or sex. It is a biological experience of God. God is no longer a theory nor an abstraction. Breathing properly brings Spirit into the body in a way that cleans and nourishes the body.

At the time the book was published, only the most courageous professionals would try it. Today, it has become so popular and socially acceptable that few professionals will admit that they haven't done it.

Rebirthing is such a good thing that I proceeded carefully, to keep the movement free of greed, and I trained so many self-employed, free, independent teachers that no one could stop the teaching, not even the government. Since conscious breathing is a spiritual purification technique, it has a natural tendency to raise people's motivation. Since it is an invisible power and it takes genuine love and intuition to produce good results in guiding a student's breathing rhythm, it has a tendency to remain a pure spiritual movement. Divine energy *is* divine, and people working with it on a daily basis get transformed by it.

On the other hand, people may try to corrupt anything. But the corruption of breathing has a tendency to be painful and too much effort. That is, when breathing is done incorrectly it produces too much discomfort and therefore is hard to "sell." Spiritual experiences are richest in the presence of a pure person. This is always true. Therefore, it is easy for a pure person to be successful.

Rebirthing is international. It is the most popular growth movement in countries like Holland and Poland. It has gone more slowly in India, because breathing yogas have been taught continually over the centuries and people in India are less inclined to get excited about something they are familiar with, even if they haven't experienced the full power of breathing.

By far the most exciting thing that has happened to me and the other breathers who know about Him, is the conscious awareness of the presence of Babaji in the world. There are many great gurus and even immortal yogis in the world, but there is only one supreme manifestation of God in human form and this is Babaji.

The idea of God the Eternal Father in a human body is almost too outrageous to conceive. That he is alive and available in the twentieth century is mind fracturing. Babaji has the ability to materialize and dematerialize a human body, to come and go on planet earth as he pleases. It is more difficult to write about Babaji than breathing. I have put more information about him in my new book *Physical Immortality, The Science of Everlasting Life,* published by Celestial Arts.

To be in Babaji's presence is the ultimate growth experience. Babaji is the most beautiful human being on planet earth. Seeing him in the flesh and talking with him is the greatest human experience that we are capable of. Babaji is the teacher and the power source of Moses, Elijah, Melchizedek, Jesus and all other world

Saviors. Babaji is the Creator of the universe who takes responsibility to set it right when it gets too far off course. He returns in human form when our human drama and our planet is in great danger. He is the answer to our prayers. Babaji has come many times, but people ignorant of the Bible and especially the Indian scriptures have no knowledge of him.

To take the time and money to visit him while he is here is the greatest gift you can give yourself. If enough people visit Babaji, we will have peace on earth and one human family.

It is obvious why he is here. The U.S. government spends over 60 percent of its billion-dollar budget on death machines and cuts back on helping the poor. The destruction of World Wars I and II were not enough to teach us. The life energy of human beings has gotten so weak that our materialism has made us into machines. The truly human qualities are so weak that we prefer to spend our money on death instead of life.

Babaji's message of the true religion is truth, simplicity and love. Material things have to be taken care of. Most people are in bondage, slaves to their material possessions. Are we unable to take time for peace?

The purpose of Babaji's physical presence in the world is to improve the quality of human energy and intelligence. Babaji imparts his life energy through the simple yoga methods of earth, air, water, fire and mind purification. Rebirthing is about air and water purification. Since this book was published I have added earth and fire practices to my teaching. Fasting, manual labor, and meditation on a fire can also clean the energy body. (For more information see my physical immortality book. There is a one-page summary in the back.

This *Rebirthing in the New Age* book is now a historical classic, but it is still so relevant that its future as a bestseller is only now becoming possible. We will see. Some books mirror change. Some books cause change. This book is the latter. Although the loving work of thousands of breathing guides are the true cause of this change, this book has been a valuable tool. It has inspired people to try the breathing lessons, it has instructed the teachers and improved the quality of their work, it has helped the students avoid many, many problems. It may still be a book of the future, but it is helping to cause and create this future.

The political and economic ideas in this book are still visionary. People seem to require a certain amount of spiritual enlightenment, personal purification, and prosperity before they are willing to be socially concerned.

There is much I would like to change and add to this new edition, but it is already valuable as it is. By the time you have learned and practiced and integrated the ideas in this book, perhaps we will have finished more advanced books for you.

I maintain a full-time training center called Campbell Hot Springs and Consciousness Village in Sierraville, California. Here we have up-to-date information about all these ideas. This is my main home.

In rereading the book for the revision, I noticed how vague the word *rebirthing* is. The word rebirthing was originally used because we used redwood hot tubs to stimulate birth memories and people literally rewrote their birth scripts in the subconscious. A hot tub is a simulated womb. The early rebirthers became birth trauma specialists. We watched thousands of people relive their birth experience and learned more about the psychophysical implications of birth on human behavior than any people on earth.

After a year of experimenting, I learned that breathing is not only the focal point of birth, but is the primary vehicle of restoring divine energy into the human mind and body. So rebirthing primarily means the rehabilitation of breathing. Rebirthing is more descriptively called *conscious breathing* or *energy breathing*. Rebirthing is primarily a relaxed continuous breathing rhythm in which the inhale is connected to the exhale in a continuous circle. This rhythm has to be intuitive, because the purpose of the breathing is to breathe life energy as well as air. Breathing life energy cannot be done with a mechanical breathing technique. Energy is the source of the physical body and the universe. The breathing mechanism is a vehicle to reach aliveness, but it is not automatic. Spiritual breathing is intuitive, it is an inspiration, not a discipline. The key to success at conscious breathing is softness and gentleness.

Sondra uses the word *rebirth* with at least two other meanings. One is to refer to any energy experience or change which can be either a physical or spiritual energy. The other one is to refer to a significant emotional transformation brought about by insights, new thoughts, and understanding of life and oneself. These four definitions of the word, rebirth, may help you to understand this book.

In addition to these definitions, Babaji sometimes calls it an American form of Pranayama. In spite of the fact that I called it conscious breathing now, people still sometimes have a "16mm movie" of their own birth on the first session.

It is necessary to clarify that Abubabaji and Babaji are two different persons. Abubabaji is a great yogi whom we met in 1977. Babaji is the eternal manifestation of God in human form who directs the universe and the evolution of the human family.

Abubabaji has healed as many as five thousand people in one day. Babaji of course is the source of all healing. Until you have actually met Babaji in his physical body and experienced his omniscience, his eternal and divine presence, it may be difficult to conceive of such a possibility. But he is a reality. He has lived time and again in Herakhan Village since the earth was created. This fact has been published over and over again for thousands of years in the Indian Scriptures.

Enjoy the original.

Enjoy the additions.

Truth, Simplicity and Love,

Leonard Orr
Box 234
Sierraville, CA 96126

OVERCOMING THE FEAR OF LETTING PEOPLE KNOW THAT I AM NOW AND FOR THE MOST PART ALWAYS HAVE BEEN TOTALLY DEVOTED TO GOD JUST LIKE YOU ARE—EVEN THOUGH WE MAY NOT THINK SO FROM TIME TO TIME OR IT MAY NOT LOOK IT TO THE NEIGHBORS
or
HOW TO GET OUT OF YOUR HEAD BY SAYING WHAT YOU REALLY MEAN

Sondra has asked me to tell you that one of the original titles to this personal statement was "Help—I'm in the Self-Improvement Business," but my life has changed so much in the past twenty-four hours alone that this title is no longer appropriate or necessary. This morning, for example, I saw Abubabaji for the first time. I went to the airport to see him off. Immediately afterwards, when I went to the parking lot, I was overcome by feelings . . . and at last I knew what I really wanted to say here.

This book is about many very beautiful ideas and the ordinary and very beautiful people that share them with each other and with the world. These people think of themselves as the Theta Community, though there are really no boundaries as far as I can see. I have been associated with this community since its start and so Sondra asked me to make a contribution to the book. I am both honored and grateful that she has been so patient with me as I struggled to find the words for what is in my heart. I believe the struggle is ended.

I used to be a very evasive talker. If I didn't have the answers, I could think them up on the spot—and thus I knew it all. I used to hide a lot behind my answers. But, when I tried repeatedly to write this article I could really see there would be no more hiding, there would perhaps be no more need for hiding. It's not that I don't care what people think . . . and feel . . . it's just that I have found out at last that I care about what I think and feel . . . and want to express. And I have found after intensive searching that there is really only one thing I want to say.

I just want to say that I am totally grateful to God that he has led me to these people . . . and that I am totally thankful to Him for everything I have experienced in my life.

And to each of you I would like to say—I love you. Thank you so much for being alive.

I hope this message makes some sense because before—and it seems an eternity ago now—nothing did. God bless you.

At last I am speechless.

Bill Chappelle

My First Rebirth, 1974
Sondra Ray

Dear Mother,

Well, Mom, I finally outdid everything I have ever done! I have just had the highest experience of my life—I have found ecstacy, and I'm staying there most of the time! It actually beats the University of Florida, my wedding, my life in the Andes, the trip on the Amazon, crossing the Beagle Straits, getting free in Hungary, living in Hawaii, taking LSD, and even orgasm! Remember all *those* letters? Well, this one will blow your mind. I was RE-BIRTHED, and I mean that literally. I just got "exorcised" from my birth trauma in a redwood hot tub.

It all began when I decided to go on a retreat with Leonard Orr. I had to take off work for a week, and my only regret is that I told them I was doing it because you were sick. Well, how could I tell them that I wanted time to handle my birth trauma? Two weeks ago I had shown the obstetricians at work Dr. LeBoyer's *Birth Without Violence* and they told me it was hogwash.

Anyway, we rented a secluded place called Venture Lodge in the mountains near Santa Cruz. I was the first one to arrive Friday night. It was not quite dark and the mist was rolling over the place, covering the lodge and the swimming pool, which was out in the middle of a meadow. At the end of the pool was a sunken redwood hot tub, the steam rising from it to join the mist. The place looked eerie. I couldn't find anyone, yet the door to the lodge was open, the fireplace was going and there was incense burning. It was as if some Kundalini Yoga group had been there. I stretched out on the pillows, which were everywhere. A caretaker appeared and told me the place used to be a nudist camp. I wondered what he would think if he knew what we were about to do . . . however, he looked ready for anything.

The other fifteen people Leonard had invited began to appear. We all sat by the fire drinking hot chocolate and waiting for him. (I think he was late on purpose so that all our fears would come up. They did!) I was relieved when he walked in and started a little talk. He reviewed for us the effects of the birth trauma: the shock we all experienced coming from that safe, watery environment— the bliss of the womb—out into the atmosphere; how it was like landing on the moon without preparation. Also, how our bodies were unnecessarily tortured (being held upside down, for instance) because most doctors and mothers are "plugged into" their *own* birth traumas. How the fear and pain at birth stay in the depths of our minds all our lives and have a negative impact on us daily. And about the negative generalizations we made then, and how all these things have created "the universe is against me" syndrome.

Well, I was ready to get on with it. I wanted that tension and suppressed grief out of my body. I would have gone into the tub right then, but Leonard told us "No." Our "assignment" was to go to bed and stay there until mid-afternoon of the next day. He wanted us to become "activated" or to begin to induce the memory of our births, since we tend to re-create the womb every day in bed and subliminally re-experience our birth traumas every time we wake up! At eleven the next morning, I was feeling very claustrophobic in my sleeping bag. I asked Leonard if I could please get out. He said "No." The last couple of hours I was feeling something of what Dr. Grof from Czechoslovakia calls "no-exit terror" in the womb.

We finally began, around two in the afternoon. Fifteen of us sat around the hot tub apprehensively. I watched the first of us, Elana, enter the tub, float face down with snorkel and nose plug, and start breathing. It sounded very loud. Leonard sat in a chair looking down at her. I was not sure what kind of psychic trip he was doing, but I knew it was *something* for sure. For some strange reason, I soon was overwhelmed with sadness. But before I had time to cry, Elana suddenly leaped out of the tub and landed in my lap, writhing in pain. I was frozen. I could not move any part of my body. It was the first time in all my years of nursing that I didn't know instantly what to do. Even if I had known, I couldn't have moved. It was awful.

Everyone else responded similarly. We were like helpless infants. None of us could speak—except for Leonard. Elana was terrified, and Leonard came to help her. Somehow he soon had her smiling and laughing. I was confused, very confused.

I was going slightly unconscious, or something. All I knew was that my rebirth was to follow Fred's. By the time he got in the tub, I was a mess. I just looked at him and started to cry. Suddenly I rolled up in a ball on the deck near the tub. I was sobbing hysterically, not then aware that I was beginning my rebirth without even having entered the tub. I could hear my own crying. It did not sound like me at all. It sounded like a newborn wailing in torment.

My sadness seemed unlimited. I asked someone to take my clothes off; I couldn't stand the scorching feeling of them against my skin. After a long time I finished crying and told Leonard I still wanted to go in the tub. But they had to lift me in; I was helpless. By that time, I couldn't even manage the snorkel (and me, a scuba diver). I sank to the bottom. I guess I stayed there for ages. (Later they told me everyone was worried about me, except Leonard.) I finally came up for some air. Somebody was holding me then.

Suddenly I started breathing very fast. I was bursting. I couldn't get enough air, it seemed, even though I was breathing very fast. I couldn't figure anything out. I felt that I could *never* stop that fast breathing. It overtook me. Something was breathing me! Somewhere in there something very deep in me started welling up. It was heavy, it was dark and it was growing. I couldn't stop it; it took over my whole body. A scream came out of me. I wasn't scared any more.

I told them, "There's more." I breathed out more and more and more of . . . I don't know what. I felt them carry me out and gently lay me down. I began to tingle all over. It kept building and spreading. It felt like a thousand orgasms! I began to throw my head from side to side wildly, in joy. My neck was totally loose for the first time. I heard someone say, "Her joy is just infectious." Tears were rolling down my cheeks. I had never felt that happy in my life . . . never. I heard the breeze totally, all of it, it seemed, though I hadn't noticed any breeze before. I heard the trees talk to me.

Suddenly I wanted real music. I wanted a celebration. I wanted singing. I asked Leonard if I could have Jan sing for me. Maybe, I thought, she would be willing to play some of the songs she had played on her guitar by the fire the night before. Leonard sent someone into the woods to find her. (She has astral-projected, I thought!) Suddenly Jan was there beside me playing my very favorite song, the one I wanted but couldn't request because I didn't remember the name. I wept again. I had *never* heard anything so beautiful.

And then they carried me to the Rolfing table in the middle of the sunny meadow. I still had not opened my eyes. John pressed on my body gently and the ecstasy was so great, I floated. I was above the trees. I suddenly realized I was having an out-of-body experience. I wondered if he could tell. And then he said, "Well, Sondra, there is no point in working on your body if you are not in it." How did he know? What was all this telepathy going on? When I got back in my body it was just as good, so I stayed in. It seemed like the first time I had ever entered my body totally. It was a new experience to be in it totally like that. And I loved my body more than I ever thought possible.

So I told John, "I am going to open my eyes now," as if I knew it was going to be something special. I didn't feel funny about announcing it like that. What I saw was a real spectacle. I actually "saw" all the electrons in the universe at once, all the particles in the air, and all of it was sparkling. And then I began to see the trees. They were vibrating many colors of green that I had never seen before. Oh, Mother, it was magic!

I felt overwhelming love for everyone there. I asked John to lie down next to me. I wanted to hold someone, to hug someone. I was walking on air for the rest of the retreat. When we came home, ·my mind was preoccupied with getting back in a tub. Yesterday I tried it again. But I'll tell you about that another time. Right now I just want to tell everyone to try this. And I want to tell you how much I thank you for letting me be born at home on the kitchen table. I am so glad nobody took me away from you after my birth; I needed you there and you comforted me.

Happy Mother's Day! (Isn't it interesting I did it at this time?)

I love you,

Sondra

PART I

The Story of Theta

1 The Beginning

Shortly after I had done *est* (Erhard Seminar Training) in San Francisco I had a car accident. Nothing serious. I just backed into something and smashed up my Fiat. The peculiar thing was, I was doing this about once a month. I couldn't seem to stop. I ran into poles, hydrants, old trucks—you name it. It was costing me a fortune to keep my car in repair. I was about to hire a chauffeur and quit driving. At an *est* graduate seminar after the accident I burst into tears. Two concerned men sitting nearby listened as I poured out my story of the accidents and my feelings of desperation.

"Don't worry, Sondra," they comforted me. "We'll take you to Leonard Orr."

"Who is that?" I wanted to know. "What can he do?"

"Oh, he will clear you up on that, and much more," they said rather mysteriously. I was intrigued.

The very next day my two new friends drove me to a gorgeous country home in Woodside, fifty miles south of San Francisco. About thirty-five people were seated on the grass under the trees which surrounded the house. A man stood before them holding a chart with some circles and dots on it. He was diagramming the mind. It was Leonard Orr.

I soon found myself absolutely awestruck by his ideas. All the missing links in my life began to come clear. Things really made sense. "Once you get this," he commented, "you will get hooked on it." Little did I know! During a break I wandered up to him and said something trivial, just to be talking to him. Before I knew it, he had out his appointment book and I was signing up for a private session with him—which was, of course, exactly what I had wanted.

Over the next few days I grew excited each time I reviewed my notes from Leonard's talk. I became obsessed with sharing this new knowledge. Inviting my best friend Susan out for breakfast, I went over every line I had taken down during the seminar. Susan is brilliant, and I figured if she was impressed, then I must be on to something. She loved it. I felt elated. My mind kept saying, "At last! Here is the total truth about life!"

I prepared for my private session with Leonard by writing down all my hangups and my urgent questions. I walked into his apartment, handed him the paper, and sat down. He started reading it without a word, making me feel quite comfortable about having done it that way. I had made a long list, and Leonard dispensed with the items one by one. The solutions came so fast I wondered where my mind had been all my life. Where had *he* been all my life?

When he came to my car-wrecking syndrome, Leonard merely gave me a sentence to write: "I now have a safe driving consciousness."

"What?" I responded. "Is that all?"

"Yes," he said. "But you must write it at least ten times a day." He explained that the sentence he had given me was an *affirmation,* that is, a positive thought which you choose to immerse in your consciousness to produce a desired result.

I didn't quite believe this would work, so I deliberately chose a far-fetched example. "Do you mean to say," I wanted to know, "I could even get men to call me on the telephone using affirmations?"

"Of course," he replied. "Try it." Then he told me to write: "I now receive an abundant inflow of calls from men when I am at home." I had always had a certain nervousness about telephones which began when my father was an engineer with the telephone company. He died when I was young and I apparently concluded that telephones had something to do with death. I always managed to be out when men called me—especially men I cared about.

Naturally, I worked on the phone affirmation first! I wrote it for about four days, ten times a day. I couldn't believe what happened. All my old lovers began to call me, men I had not heard from for months, some for years. I decided then to see how far I could go with this affirmation and continued to write it for several days more. Incredible as it sounds, I began to receive telephone calls during the night, wrong numbers from strange men.

Somewhat embarrassed, I returned to Leonard and told him I had apparently overdone it. "You must reverse this thing. I can't sleep," I exclaimed. So he gave me a new affirmation: "I now receive telephone calls only from the men I want to hear from." That worked too. I was then willing to go ahead with the car affirmation. I have not wrecked my car since!

I started to go to all Leonard's seminars. He was getting to be very much in demand, so my next appointment with him was at midnight! I went there to handle what he calls a "personal law"—your most dominant negative consciousness factor. He was heading for Carmel, and told me to write some things down while he packed. I followed him from room to room trying to hear what he was telling me. Suddenly he proposed that I drive him to Carmel, saying I could have my consultation free if I did. I couldn't resist, and didn't even consider how far it was and that I had to be at work in San Francisco early the next day. I finished writing three things I liked about my father, three things I disliked about my father, etc. Then we got in my little Fiat and he read it all by the map light.

I proceeded to analyze myself. "Well, Leonard, it is obvious. I married my father."

"Oh, yes?" He was amused. "Well, what about . . ." and he laid out a wholly different analysis. My mind seemed to be made of putty all of a sudden. He had nailed me. How could he possibly have figured me out from one crummy piece of paper that said nothing? What do you say to such a man? Was he real? Then I relaxed. There was no other way to handle it because he started commenting on my thoughts second by second.

"Leonard, this is ridiculous. If you are going to read my thoughts like that we won't even have to talk."

"Yes, won't that be great? We can just sit here and pass thoughts back and forth."

In Carmel, we entered a house and found a beautiful woman named Efale. I liked her immediately. She seemed surprised to see Leonard. I wondered what it was all about, but I was tired and I had to leave again in a couple of hours. Leonard wakened me at five and saw me off. He was incredibly gentle, incredibly loving and caring. I was very "high" as I drove home after being in his presence.

Shortly thereafter I went to Europe. Before I left I decided to test the affirmation thing one more time. I had limited money for the trip to Vienna and Budapest, and I decided I would try to save by not paying for food. I thought maybe I could set it up somehow so I wouldn't have to buy any of my meals. I wrote an affirmation to that effect. The results were awesome. People continually treated me to dinner on the trip. I did not have to buy myself one single meal. When I got back home from Europe I was eager to call Leonard and acknowledge this miracle, but decided to wait until early the next morning.

During the night I had a dream: In the dream I was trying to find Leonard. I went to the *est* office and looked everywhere. He was not there. I asked people where he was. People kept looking for him behind various doors. Every door they opened revealed someone else. I finally became angry.

"Where is the real Leonard Orr?" I protested. Someone finally said to me, "Leonard is no longer on the *est* staff."

In the morning I called Leonard. "Leonard, I am back from Europe. What has been happening?"

"I am no longer on the *est* staff," he commented. I was struck by the way the words came out exactly as in my dream.

"When did this happen?" I asked.

"Late last night," he said.

I told him about my dream. After that, our real friendship began.

One afternoon I sat in an astrology seminar wondering what on earth I was doing there, since I certainly did not believe the stars control me. But something had brought me there that day. As I mused over it, Leonard entered the room from the back, talking all the way up the aisle. Was there anyone in the room, he wanted to know, who wished to move into his new house, a huge old Victorian? I found my hand going up, even before he reached the front of the room, even before I realized that I had no plans to move, even before I remembered we hardly knew each other. I was very confused. My friend Susan had said she thought I would be moving soon. How did she know, and not me? I also wondered how Leonard could just walk into a room and ask for house mates. What did he know about us that would lead him to take such a chance?

I knew that Leonard had started in the self-improvement business in 1968. Before that he had worked at various sales jobs. One day he realized that the easiest way to become wealthy was to do what he enjoyed doing most—which was to stay home and read metaphysical books. As an experiment, he stayed home two and a half days a week for a month to work on improving the quality of his ideas. He actually tripled his income as a salesman by staying home more. A number of his clients became interested in the ideas he was exploring and they paid him to stay home and read, so he could tell them what he learned and they could improve the quality of their thoughts. It was a remarkable confirmation of his intuitive theory. As a result, his clients doubled their incomes.

I used to wonder why everyone couldn't see Leonard the way I did. It never occurred to me that they were probably expecting some kind of Eastern-looking guru. Leonard is not like that at all. He often dresses sloppily, wearing weird colors and scuffed shoes. He breathes heavily with great sighs and people often react to this by assuming he is bored. He talks in a low tone and sometimes his listeners get so relaxed that they go to sleep. There is no commotion when he enters a room. People don't stand up and applaud or anything. He is just like anyone else at his own seminars. He looks ordinary.

Without really understanding why I was doing it, I soon stood with this both ordinary and extraordinary man on the sidewalk at 301 Lyon Street, San Francisco, staring up at a huge old house that seemed to go on forever. Leonard explained that it was to be the headquarters of Theta Seminars. Theta is the greek letter which is a circle with a line crossing it; for him Theta symbolized infinite being manifesting on a material level. My strongest impressions of that first tour of the house have to do with mirrors and fireplaces. Leonard was excited about the marble bathroom. He suggested that I take the room adjoining his bedroom, but that did not seem appropriate to me. I recognized by then that he was more to me than a potential lover.

Meeting again at the big house that evening, we flopped all our belongings on the floor, since there wasn't any furniture at all. The house echoed. Thirty rooms of spirits? I wondered. The vibrations were very strange. We didn't stay long that first night. The whole thing seemed a little strange, but I still did not question my intuition in any way.

In the empty dining room the next morning, we began to unpack. Leonard suddenly noticed that one of the wooden panels had been removed from the dining room wall.

"It wasn't like that last night," he pointed out to me.

"I know," I said, while reaching inside to see what might be there. Nothing but space. I wondered what had been hidden there and who had gotten in, and how. We began to roam through the mansion looking for doors or windows that might give us clues. Everything was tightly shut.

"There must be a secret entrance," I concluded. I told Len I was going outside to check around. Outside I realized that we had moved into a strange neighborhood; we were on the edge of Haight-Ashbury. It had not occurred to me earlier. Our house was painted so brightly and took up so much of the block that I had never even noticed the run-down houses alongside. Next to us was a kind of falling-apart house which was actually a Black Baptist Church—on the bottom floor, that is. I wandered over to it as a girl came downstairs. She seemed to be high on something, and looked as if she had been sleeping in her clothes for ten days. She was extremely friendly.

"Say," I put out, "did you happen to see anyone crawling in any windows next door last night?"

"No," she said flatly, "but I used to live there so I can tell you all about the place." She proceeded to take me on a tour of my new home. It was a crash pad, she said, a drug pushing center, a home for drug addicts and I don't know what all. She began to point out all the drug hiding places and commented that obviously someone had seen the new tenants and come back to get the last hidden "stashes." I suspected *her*, but what did it matter now? She showed me how boards collapsed behind the fireplaces, how the floor had loose slats which could be removed, how ladders led to hidden roofs behind chimneys, how laundry chutes led to other places, and so on. I was intrigued and found myself hanging on her every word. Finally she stopped in her tracks and pulled up her shirt, proudly showing me a huge scar on her abdomen. "I was a Zebra victim," she boasted.

Was *she* going to be my new neighbor? Was this where I was going to live? Was Leonard going to turn *this* into a higher consciousness center? Was all this real? She noticed then how "straight" I was, and we parted.

Leonard took the big bedroom facing the panhandle of Golden Gate Park—he liked the trees and the fireplace—and by that time he had a possible candidate for the little room adjoining his. To me, she was ravishingly beautiful. She was Eve, the maiden, the mother, the goddess, the queen all in one. They were perfect, I thought. I was thrilled with the idea of her being in the house. On her first visit, however, she seemed uncertain. Leonard was certain. He ordered her a special new bed. I remember thinking it was kind of a fairy tale . . . she left for Europe and this new bed was waiting for her to return. Nobody could sleep in it; she had to be the first one. So there was this room with the bare box spring and mattress, waiting.

I picked a two-room suite where, according to Miss Zebra Victim, thirty people once had crashed. Actually it was one tall room with an adjoining room that was all windows and faced the street. The view was terrible, and it was crazy because I had to put my bed in front of a window that led to somebody else's room.

Leonard informed me that an older woman was moving in, an artist. I was reluctant to accept her because she reminded me of my mother, but I decided to try. She chose the room alongside mine. Unfortunately, the door was missing between our rooms. She would get up at 5 A. M., turn the light on and paint. I became increasingly uncomfortable about her.

One day Leonard started installing a redwood tub in our own basement. It was the first piece of furniture we had, besides our beds. Leonard seemed in a great hurry for the tub builders to get it done. They often worked through the night. Meanwhile I went about my business of nursing, leaving every morning at 7:30 for the hospital and getting home every afternoon at 5:30. I never really considered the implications of having a rebirthing tub in my own basement. In fact, I just didn't go down there. There were so many basement rooms and it was eerie. I started avoiding the whole idea. My first few rebirths had been so powerful that I was becoming a little afraid to go on.

* * * * * *

Back in San Francisco, about a week after the first rebirth experience, most of us were ready to try it again. So Leonard piled us in a car and took us to the home of a friend who had a lovely outdoor hot tub.

Elana went first again, and this time I was able to stay more conscious during her rebirth. I was preparing to "catch her" once again as lovingly as I could. Only this time she crawled out by herself, and kept right on crawling all over the deck. Leonard let her do this as long as she wanted, which seemed like a long time. She looked like a six-month-old baby.

Then I got in the tub. I breathed and breathed. I went back to the womb. Suddenly I was aware of someone else besides Leonard. This person's vibrations felt very heavy to my then-supersensitive body. I couldn't stand it. I became furious. It felt like a man and I hated his intrusion. Rage swept through me as I surfaced and yelled, "Someone else is in my womb! Get him out!"

I was shocked at my own anger. I am almost never in touch with anger and I just couldn't believe I was yelling. Neighbors were apparently coming out the windows. I recall Leonard saying I would have to go inside if I was going to carry on like that. Suddenly I was lying on a mat and Elana was next to me. "Thank God," I remember thinking. She seemed to be saying all the right things. She kept me talking by asking all the right questions. It was such a relief.

I was very confused. I couldn't tell if I was a baby girl or a baby boy. "Oh, my father really wanted a boy," I told her. "I can really feel his disappointment. It's awful." I cried and cried. "I'll never be good enough to please him." I didn't know it then, but I had just verbalized my own personal law.

Later I came to see that my problem in life had been over-identification with my father. I would do *anything* to please him, including subconsciously becoming a "boy." And although later on I developed an obviously feminine body, I had a great deal of male consciousness. In fact, subsequently I had to go through a kind of mental sex change. I never had homosexual desires, but I did have quite a bit to work out in becoming a complete woman.

Becoming a sex therapist was, I know now, a way of doing this. Before rebirthing I had no idea why I had relationships that were competitive with men. I didn't realize that I had gotten A's all through graduate school to please my father. Of course none of it worked. Nothing *could* work until I learned to change my personal law that I would never be good enough.

There were positive and negative aspects of my personal law, as there are with everything in the universe. The positive side of my personal law was that it did make me a very strong woman. The negative aspect was a subtle desire to compete with and intimidate men.

I was thrilled with the results of my second rebirth. Imagine going back so far that you can get in touch with what you were thinking at the moment you were born! Imagine being able to know what other people in the room were thinking at your birth! I really got excited. And then I got scared.

It took me quite a number of weeks to integrate the effects of my first two rebirths. My life seemed to be changing too fast. I walked around the house in a funk. I was not used to experiencing anger of any kind. It frightened me. Everyone in the house seemed to be a psychological mess. I told myself that because of my job it was too great a risk to try rebirthing again. But I began to feel more and more crazy. One night I asked Leonard for a consultation; we met at a restaurant called The Haven. He was goofing off with me and I got angry. I told him to at least give me some affirmations, so he wrote on a page: "Nobody loves me but Leonard so he must be crazy." I became enraged, but I didn't know it.

Driving home through the Haight, he suddenly said, "Start screaming." I froze. "What?" "Start screaming," he ordered again. I couldn't.

"Your anger is wiping me out," he protested. "If you don't scream, I will." I was aghast at what he was saying, but I couldn't scream.

So he did just what he said he would. He started screaming. I couldn't believe it. I pulled the car to the curb and began to cry. My guru was screaming. My world had come apart. It was impossible. I couldn't take it. Leonard suddenly left the car, abandoning me. That did it! I hated him. I started screaming at him. All my anger came out. I wanted to kill him. In a bit, he came around to the driver's window and gently kissed me. "Feel better now?" he wanted to know. He seemed to have known what he had to do. Leaving me was the turning point. The next day I came out of my mental fog and headed for the basement. I was ready to handle the rest of my birth trauma.

* * * * * *

Leonard's new girl friend came back from Europe. She looked ravishingly beautiful, as always. I wondered if she would settle for such a small room. She lasted one night—moved in one night and moved out the next.

I was still trying to get used to the woman in the room next to mine. She was probably all right, but I had her "set up" as my mother. It just didn't work. Then a young musician named Jim moved in. He was nice looking, sandy-haired, pleasant; but he took the room which had the window behind my bed. We immediately had to deal with problems of privacy.

One day Diane Greenleaf came to live at Theta House. She took the room next to Leonard's. Her room always emitted this special kind of smoke—like a very strange incense. When I finally went in to see it, I was amazed. She had an altar, bells, percussion instruments and all kinds of meditation oddities. I thought it was very weird until I learned about Arica. Diane always seemed like she was in a fog. And she never worked. She never *had* worked either, something which the rest of us soon had to deal with. She was a rich hippie. She had lots of time and we finally talked her into doing the grocery shopping. But everything she brought home was exotic; none of us liked it much, but we didn't want to do the shopping, either.

So we finally faced the fact that we had to create a weekly house meeting. The first one was held in the living room (somebody had lent us a couch by then—which looked pretty lost in the space of that huge room). We spent the entire meeting arguing about *when* we would have weekly house meetings. We never did come to an agreement.

I kept trying to get through to Diane, without too much luck. One day it dawned on me that she was "stoned" twenty-four hours a day. The only person who seemed to understand her was another Arican named Fred Sharpe. I first met him in the astrology seminar. He sat at the piano and did some incredible music. It was out of this world. I walked by him and he said, "What sign are you?" "Virgo," I replied. He nodded and suddenly went into a sort of trance. I wondered if he would ever come out of it. Then he played music for Virgo. It was incredible. He would close his eyes when he played as if he were getting the music from another planet, another lifetime. Later he explained this was true. He began to drop by our house a lot to see Diane, especially after we were given a piano. He always wore outrageous clothes that were never ironed. He especially liked old velvet and satin, worn with old canvas shoes and his shirt unbuttoned to the waist.

He gave wonderful concerts and people flocked to hear him. Whenever I had a "family dinner" night, he would always show up one second before we ate, even though I never called him to let him know. Those were wonderful nights that helped us all to become very close.

About that time, Elana moved in. I had met her before on a retreat and knew she was powerful. She had started Theta by organizing the seminars for Leonard in Palo Alto. I was afraid of her. It seemed to me that she talked loudly and dressed badly (her belly hung out below her blouse). Before long, I felt I couldn't stand being in the same room with her. She became the one I openly resented. I had no idea I was working out our sibling rivalry. Elana started doing rebirths in the basement, Leonard turning most of it over to her while he travelled. She brought a big change in the house. Often screams from the rebirthings could be heard throughout the house on all floors. Since we didn't have much furniture yet, the echoes seemed to go on forever. At that time we were just learning how to handle people's suppressed fears from birth and we had not quite resolved how to let go of the trauma without the noisy expression of it.

The office was right above the basement tub. This seemed to overstimulate the secretaries. One cried every day for two entire months. I was watching all of this, not knowing that I was just as much a helpless infant as the rest of them.

Meanwhile, Leonard continued to give his seminars, the best one of which he called the One-Year Seminar. Its purpose was to deal with and eradicate the "five biggies" (the birth trauma, the unconscious death urge, specific negatives, the parental disapproval syndrome, and other lifetimes). This group of about fifty met once a month in the large room on the top floor of the house. Leonard also did smaller seminars on money, self-analysis, and spiritual psychology. I went to them all over and over again.

And so it went as we processed our own psychological problems. What we were going through did turn away some business from seminars and consultations, but not all. It didn't keep people from benefiting from the house, however. In a way it was a blessing that there were problems. It prevented our growing too large, too fast and having too many people around to deal with effectively. As it was, for a long time only Leonard and Elana were able to help others. They felt it was necessary for more of us to be able to help people. Leonard was assisting each of us to become strong; he was building a "multiple guru system" which he feels is the solution for New Age living. It took us about a year to get ourselves well enough integrated to help him run Theta Seminars effectively.

In the meantime, Elana continually belched in the halls and yelled in the shower. I was trying to run the house, and it seemed to me that it was always Elana who left trails of litter behind her. I complained to her regularly, yet the more I did, the worse it got. I realize now how much she served me by giving me the opportunity to get angry without losing her love. I also had no idea how being a rebirther was affecting her—not until later when I became one, too.

Every Wednesday morning at seven I would drag everyone out of bed for a house meeting. Sometimes I got embarrassed about going into Leonard's room. I never knew which woman would be there beside him. And I would always have to get past being upset about how messy his room was. It was just a disaster . . . unpacked boxes everywhere, a too-small plaid blanket thrown on his king-size bed without a bedspread, no curtains, piles of little knick-knacks that people had given him, some of which were downright corny, and stacks of unanswered letters and unfiled papers. Often he wouldn't get up, even though he told me he definitely wanted to be at the house meetings. When he wouldn't come downstairs we had to move the meeting right into his room. We would stretch out on the bed or floor and carry on while his lady visitor would continue to sleep through it all. Leonard would vote on things with his eyes closed. This would drive me nuts because I never was sure if he heard what we were voting on or not. He would drift off to sleep and I would punch him a little. We never made much progress at those meetings.

It wasn't until Edwin moved in that we finally got things settled. Edwin had answered Leonard's ad for someone to run a political project. Len had the candidates spend the day together on the top floor; and at the end of the day he had *them* vote on which person was best. Edwin won. When he moved in, my first impression was that he looked like an organ grinder. I had no idea he was so incredibly talented, because I had always thought anybody who would walk around with holes in his shirt and a filty bathrobe must be a dunce. It took me weeks to get past all that.

Edwin chose a little room off the kitchen which was, to me, unspeakable. There was no heat and the floor was slanting. The only view from the back was a junky yard. His only view from the front was the top of the garage where the dogs shit. It was too depressing to me and I couldn't go into his room for a long time. But Edwin started cooking incredible family dinners on a very low budget. He really began winning my heart. I was delighted when he took over the shopping. He was Diane's opposite number. He would buy things at the very cheapest price and take a very spartan approach, hiding half of the food from us so it would last longer. This was communal living, I decided. Edwin was the only one who could make the grocery department work.

The house meetings became heated. Sometimes people would throw something down, yell, and stalk out. (We were all working out our parental disapproval syndrome at once.) Leonard would stay out of it by reading the morning newspaper, which infuriated me. Once in a while he would make a comment which seemed to dissolve everything at once; but most of the time he would just let us fight like a bunch of little kids. The issue always seemed to be who was *not* cleaning the kitchen. I knew I was; I was up at seven every morning playing mother. I was so compulsively clean it drove them all nuts. Once when I left a dirty cup out, everyone cheered and clapped. Elana and Edwin almost came to blows, screaming loudly at each other over the issue of food hiding. I finally decided that what we needed was a housekeeper.

Diane moved out and headed for India, and we have not heard from her since. Jessica, who had been working in the office, moved in to the little room next to Leonard's. She decorated it in sort of decadent art—heavy old lace, black antique things that seemed to be falling apart, and piles of old clothes which gave the room a very strange air. I was horrified. Elana had left to go on tour, and now I had to deal with someone else. The truth is that we were all into infancy—it just took different forms. Jessica cried a lot at the meetings. It seemed that whenever Leonard came around, she fell apart.

What kept me sane through all this was my new relationship with Marshall. We met four days after I began writing the affirmation that "I, Sondra, am now willing to let into my life the kind of man I desire." Marshall shortly moved into Theta House, and our relationship nourished both of us while we lived there together. He seemed like an angel to me when he would sit on our bed playing his guitar and singing beautiful songs which he had written. Soon Marshall began sharing his musical talents with others and often sang for us at the seminars. This especially pleased me because when we met he was a "closet" musician. He wrote many enlightened songs; one of the best was written for Dr. LeBoyer and is called "Welcome to the World."

Marshall and I began to rebirth each other, sometimes going down to the tub at three in the morning because we were so activated that we couldn't sleep. Once, in bed, some spontaneous primal rage came up for him and I encouraged him to yell it out, since everyone else in the house seemed to feel free about that. He did. The next morning all our plants had wilted! They weren't dry, either. So it was back to the tub in the basement.

If we ever felt any kind of argument coming on, we would head right to the tub. Often I would get in and breathe and feel pretty good in the water. Then I would come upstairs with an insatiable hunger; I would eat everything in sight and still feel hungry. Then I would think, it must be sex instead, so I would try that. But even lots of orgasms didn't begin to satisfy this deep craving. I would say to Marshall, "I just don't know what to do." Then I would find myself rolling up in a ball. Something deep inside me would well up gathering more and more power. What came out of my mouth suddenly would be something like, "I want my Daddy." Then I would cry and the intense craving would be over. Marshall would hold me until I went to sleep. Meanwhile, in his rebirthings, he would go unconscious and I would have to literally drag him out of the tub. He would constantly slip into anesthesia. We went on like this for weeks and weeks. We worked on affirmations together, finding ways of reprogramming our minds to eliminate the negative stuff that was coming up in our rebirthings. We also began rebirthing other people as a team. It was great to work that way because if one of us got wiped out, the other could take over. It worked very well, although sometimes after spending four or five hours in the tub we would have to go straight to bed.

I continued to develop my relationship with Leonard. Sometimes I would walk into the bathroom we shared and find him sitting in the bathtub with nothing but his nose above water, looking terribly shriveled, as if he had been there for hours. He never got angry with me for barging in. Once a voice from the bathtub said "Shut out the light"; it sounded as if it came from the womb—his voice was unrecognizable. I kept telling him to put a note on the door if he didn't want to be disturbed, but he never did that. Finally I concluded that if I wanted some time alone with Leonard I could head for the bathroom. Thus began our bathroom conversations. Usually I sat on the floor next to the antique tub and asked him questions about life. Often there would be a long period of silence before he would answer. I used to think he wasn't listening, then one day I realized that he was meditating on the answer. I went to him even for affirmations, which shows how dependent I was. But about this time Leonard started weaning me. It was very subtle and I was barely aware of it.

People were afraid of Leonard. They would go through all kinds of hell just meeting him in the halls. Then they would come to me and ask me what to do. "Leonard is the perfect mirror," I would explain. "You will see yourself every time. He will act out exactly what is going on with you." I liked this phenomenon, myself. I could always tell exactly where I was by seeing the reaction I got from Leonard. I did OK most of the time but I remained afraid to communicate any of my anger to him, so I would leave copious notes on his bed and run. He always read them, that was the nice thing.

Eventually I got really fed up with the way the business was going; I thought we needed some new blood. Steven, a friend from *est* days, had done some phone campaigns with me and I had been impressed with his strength and attractiveness, so I called him. He came over at once and Leonard had a brief meeting with him. Apparently he said to Steven, "Look, I am totally willing to have another guru here." Steven had never experienced this immediate total acceptance and acknowledgement and his body tingled all over, he told me later. He left in a daze, but before long he moved into Theta House. Things went well for a while. My only gripe with him was that he never made his bed and didn't change his sheets enough! I still had trouble letting go of my judgments about how people lived. I didn't understand how my own consciousness factors contributed to that whole housekeeping scene.

After an auspicious beginning, there came a time when Steven was at the height of his unconscious death urge and sabotaging Leonard's work to an incredible degree. He stopped Leonard in the hall and asked, "How long does it take to stop being a killer?" Leonard replied, "It took me ten years." Steven didn't like that answer. He replied, "I can't wait that long. I am ruining the business around here." "Well, Steven, I'll wait as long as it takes for you. I have forever," said Leonard. Since that day it has been clear to me that Leonard is willing to stay with any of us, even at the expense of Theta, no matter how long it takes for us to get our act together. He would let the whole thing go to save any one of us. Even when we were a total psychological mess and producing zero results he never asked us to "shape up or ship out." He allowed us to proceed at our own speeds. This is because he has total understanding of the unconscious death urge.

Six years after he began to seek enlightenment, Leonard had found himself becoming emotionally disturbed. After practicing the truth for six years, he wondered why things should get worse. Finally he concluded that the cause was his unconscious death urge. (His mother had died in 1956 and father in 1959 and both deaths served to activate his own death urge.) This urge was "running" him until he became willing to accept responsibility for it. The turning point came in 1967 when he went through a living death experience—he had to choose between life and death. After consciously choosing life he began to rebuild his life urges, but there were months and months where he just stayed in bed because he didn't feel like moving.

Steven was beginning to work out his unconscious death urge. He went through long periods of moving around like a snail. Sometimes I would ask him a question and there would be no answer at all. He was incredibly quiet, but he allowed me to hug him and I loved him so much. When he was right in the middle of the death urge and the birth trauma, he developed a crust all over his face that resembled the bottom of a dried-up volcano; his eye also started weeping continuously. He looked like a sad toad.

At this time there were, living in the house, Leonard, Elana, Marshall, Jessica, Steven, Edwin and me. One day I suggested we take the fractious house meetings down to the tub, and they began to be more successful. We also started doing "family" rebirths where all of us would rebirth one of the gang. These sessions were invaluable. We began to work on our money cases; we were moving from helpless infants toward becoming financially independent. We had all been "into" poverty during that period. Sometimes we all stayed in bed and cancelled everything.

One day Jessica moved out and Jan moved in. I was happy to see Jan again; she had sung to me at my first rebirth and I felt a real bond with her. But it wasn't easy for a new person to move in after most of us had cleared out so much emotional garbage. Jan got immediately activated. At times I wished I didn't have to be reminded of what I'd already been through, especially at six in the morning when she went into the bathroom and started retching. Every morning I woke up to the sound of her retching. I covered my head with a pillow. Marshall began to sleep with his headphones on. Eventually Jan worked her way through it and she stopped. Soon she began to assist in the rebirthing.

Our family was getting closer and closer. We loved to be together. By now we were making some real progress in the business and with the house. We finally got some furniture. We finished reading books like *The Primal Scream* and moved on to *Life and Teachings of the Masters of the Far East,* and others. We continued to "process out our cases," as we called it.

About this time, Leonard was beginning to recognize that hyperventilation is a significant part of the rebirthing process. We were all in the basement for a family rebirth when Steven started rebirthing right on the couch. He rolled up into a ball and said he couldn't breathe. He was in pain. Leonard kept telling him to breathe. He choked some, and began to relive his first breath. With Leonard coaching, he kept on breathing through the pain and fear, faster and faster, until somehow he "broke free" and his breathing seemed to be on a whole new level. It was his breathing release. The next day he shed his "skin" and looked years younger.

We started attracting some really great, "together" people. One who joined us was Kyle Hedon Os. He had been given another name, his father's, at birth. When his father died, Kyle decided to give up his name and start a whole new identity. To choose a name, he listed all the qualities he wanted in his new being. Then he meditated on them and waited for the universal mind to suggest a name that would embody those qualities; thus, whenever he heard his new name it would affirm in him all the traits he most wanted for himself. Kyle started a new fad at Theta and a lot of us changed all or part of our names. His seminar, "Name Changing, A New Reality," became very popular. Kyle is an excellent consultant. We went to him with big problems and always came away feeling as if our minds had been dynamited. It was funny how he started. He just showed up out of the blue one day and went from room to room offering to give a consultation for fifteen dollars. After experiencing an hour's consultation with Kyle, I told him to double his price immediately. People now pay him fifty to one hundred dollars an hour, and they always get their money's worth.

We attracted others like Lynda, Kristian, Diane and Bobby. They seemed to "get it" much faster than we had; part of the reason was that the rest of us had jettisoned enough emotional garbage that we were able to help them. The seminars were better by then, and the rebirthing was also improved. Our momentum was building with the addition of these great people to our team. We were able to start travelling; we were able to experience more prosperity; we grew up and became gurus together.

* * * * * *

It was not until a year after my first rebirth that I completed my breathing release. Constantly going in the water had kept me from it, but at first we did not know that we could do rebirthing without water; we thought it was primarily the water that created results. However, Leonard learned, after much practice, that it is the breathing that does it. So the idea of dry rebirths was born, and I flew to San Diego to participate in a special training program that Leonard was offering to teach the new technique.

Every afternoon we would do dry rebirths in groups of ten, and every morning all fifty of us would cram in one little room, body to body on the floor, and share our experiences. The intensity increased with each passing day, and by the end of the week every breath was a rebirth. I was fortunate to have two very good dry rebirths, one by Bobbie Birdsall and one by my old friend, Elana. I had also spent several long days in consultation with Kyle. By the time I got back to San Francisco I was really "psyched."

John Wright met me at the airport and took me to the Unitarian Church, where there was a sex therapists' conference at which I promoted and sold my new book, *I Deserve Love*. John seemed to like the new "space" I was in and decided to stay with me all day. But he had been sitting next to me for only fifteen minutes when he got totally "plugged in" (activated). He said, "I must go lie down." Before I knew it, I was rebirthing him right there in the church pew. It was great to know about dry rebirthing, because there surely wasn't any water around!

By midnight I felt ready for something. I wasn't sure what it would be, but instinctively I knew it would be special. John was glad to go to the basement with me, since he was feeling so appreciative of his afternoon rebirth. First I got into the hot water, so that I would be very relaxed before I tried doing a dry rebirth on myself. I breathed for a while with the snorkel, then stretched out on a Rolfing table and concentrated on breathing, consciously breathing.

Then I began playing some games with the tingling as it ran through me. The right side of my head seemed totally clear after an hour, and there was a lot of energy there. The left side seemed black and heavy. I picked out one negative thought and tried to visualize it in my left brain; then I sent some of that vibrating energy over from the right side to devour it. It worked—I could almost see the negative thoughts being eaten up! I entertained myself for ages with this. John was very patient and just lay there next to me. I relaxed more and more and the negatives got heavier and heavier. My breathing got more difficult. I kept on going, though there were many times I wanted to get up and leave. But I kept on going. And then it seemed I no longer had control of my breaths. They became smaller and smaller and shorter and shorter, until I just stopped altogether. There was no more air. I could not breathe another breath. Everything became very silent; it was like the terrible stillness before a storm. I couldn't move.

Suddenly something entered me, a breath from outside me. It started taking over, and my chest was moving very deep, very fast. There was so much air coming into me I had no idea where to put it. I felt that I was going to burst. Needing help, I yelled, "Come in, Kyle and Jesus!"

The minute I did that, everything broke. I got control of my breath. I totally let go. I went into deep, deep sobbing. Everything was released. It felt wonderful. The spirit had entered my body. I was directly with God. Rushes of divine energy came through me. A tremendous white light surrounded me. It seemed to go out thirty or more feet. It was very brilliant!

Since experiencing my breathing release I have had a lot of fun with rebirthing. Although I don't work on my own birth anymore, I still use rebirthing as a mental bath or clearing process. Once your breathing is "connected" as a result of completing the breathing release, you are forever in touch with your breath in a new way. You are able to recognize instantly when your breath is "stuck" as a result of accumulating negative mental mass. An unexpected bonus is that sex is totally new after a breathing release. Now I always rebirth myself when I make love. The more I breathe, the more love I can take in; and I can really let go because there is no longer anything buried in my consciousness that I have to fear.

I have seen rebirthing go through all the growing pains and changes necessary to make it the safe and efficient process it is today. I went from wet to dry, you might say, in my evolvement with rebirthing. Today the rebirthee will go from dry to wet. Later you will read the rebirthing history of someone who has done it the new way, as you would if you were to start tomorrow.

* * * * * *

When I moved into that big, old Victorian house I never dreamed that one day I would be leading seminars across the country and rebirthing people all around the world. When people welcome me with cheers or applause I am truly astonished. I am just being myself, you know—it is just like breathing. Does one get excited about breathing? (Well, actually one does after having experienced the healing and connectedness of the breathing release. But by now it is all integrated and natural, and I no longer think about it.) The important thing for you to know is that you can be a "star" just as easily as anyone else. We are all equally divine.

When I committed myself to working in the consciousness movement for a living, I had many doubts and fears. I was afraid to put my name on the Theta calendar. My friend, Tim, stood up at a meeting and called to me, "Well, Sondra, what are you going to call your seminar?" I was not only embarrassed, but terrified. Now I'm really going to have to do it, I thought fearfully.

The day of my first seminar I was afraid that people might actually come to it. Later I was scared that they wouldn't! At one minute before the hour, nobody had arrived, and I was both relieved and disappointed. However, in the next minute five of my friends showed up to take my seminar. I couldn't imagine why they would want to come—I am a talking seminar all the time!

They even paid me, and at first I felt guilty about that. Now I am sure of the value of what I do.

As it turned out, I was stuck on the number five for a long time; for months I never created more than five people at one of my seminars. A strong fear of disapproval was holding me back. I also was too much involved with my own case when I first started. (Even in the beginning of my larger trainings, occasionally I would need to call a break to go out and lie down on the hotel floor and rebirth myself before continuing the seminar. I just didn't know how to handle all the energy changes people go through.) Eventually I expanded my consciousness to ten people, then fifteen, and kept adding five until I reached my comfort zone of fifty. In the same way, a little at a time, I gained the confidence to write my first book. Since then, many people have told me how their lives have been transformed by participating in my Loving Relationships Training and practicing affirmations as described in *I Deserve Love.*

Most of us try to set up the game so that we have a safe place to process ourselves and be real. One of the reasons Leonard invented the One-Year Seminar was so that he would have a safe place to work out his own psychological problems. Not long ago, twenty of my Loving Relationships Training graduates rented private planes and we left for Maui, Hawaii. We rented the entire Heavenly Hana Inn for two and one-half days. I was offering an advanced training, but since this was the first one I considered it experimental. As I looked at the twenty graduates surrounding me on the floor, my love for them overwhelmed me—maybe it was their love for me that overwhelmed me. Again, they were actually willing to pay me to be there. I was honored. I wondered how it was going to work out.

The first night of the seminar everyone did a process whereby they openly communicated all their reservations about each other—they "got clean" with everyone else in the room. The room lightened up, and the love was flowing. The second day we dissolved barriers and fears to loving each other unconditionally. Some of the processes were very intense and people went right into their birth traumas (which we considered very valuable). Any time one can clear out primal trauma of birth, it is a blessing. You could really feel the "space" in the inn transform after that and we got higher and higher.

That evening we did group massages, four people massaging one person. This increased our ability to receive. We also did nude processes about loving your body. Sex was not the issue or the purpose, and fears about its turning into an orgy were dissolved. By the third day I myself was so sensitive to the love vibration in the room that I surrendered to it spontaneously and went into a state I had never been in before. I began to experience massive doses of energy coming through me. It was like having one cosmic orgasm after another.

Jesse, a quiet, super powerful man, was working on my crown chakra. I had no idea what he was doing exactly; however, my whole body went into intense pleasurable spasms. I felt so safe with the group that I did not try to stop what was happening in any way. One by one several others came to lie next to me to get a rush of the energy coming through me. As I held each person, something happened: There was a spontaneous rebirth to the point of a fast breathing release. I was carried from the couch to the bed so more people could lie next to me. At one time there were eight on the bed with me. At times there was so much love coming through me I wept unashamedly. People standing in the room fell on the floor and wept or went into a primal state. At one point someone went into an epileptic seizure. I could not rise to assist him; however, other rebirthers in the room went over and rebirthed him right through it. I knew intuitively it was a cure for him. (This I can now validate months later). It was an intense moment because many people in the room had never seen a *grand mal* seizure. At that moment all my years of nursing were useless. What worked was a rebirth. Everyone present knew they could handle anything in a rebirth situation after that. I thanked him for letting go in front of us, so we could learn the lesson in spiritual healing.

Once I strongly felt other "presences" there in the room with us, whose forms I could not see. It seemed like a scene from the Bible—everyone was glowing with white light. There is no power on earth or anywhere else stronger than love energy, and we all had a direct experience of it that day. I was very grateful that the group of loving individuals created a safe place for me to grow, and from that day I have never been quite the same. The more loving I am, the faster people get through their rebirths. Groups gathered together in a spiritual community are invaluable. Jesus said, "Where two or three are gathered together in my name, there will I be also." So don't try to do it alone; that is the hard way.

Elana is now one of the most successful women in the consciousness movement. During the past year she has traveled a great deal on the One-Year Seminar circuit. (There are now one-year seminars in major cities across the country.) She also leads rebirth trainings in many cities. Elana feels that she has found a method that will revolutionize rebirthing, bringing it to its ultimate fulfillment. She is studying the method in depth, beginning to teach it, and hopes to be able to offer the New Age the fastest, most streamlined technique to mastery of the physical universe.

She has taped seminars on many aspects of consciousness: on parent-child relationships; on the Bible, after studying it from the widened viewpoint of physical immortality; on financial freedom for women; and on love, sex and spirituality. Her main interest is in achieving total mastery and in helping others. She feels the highest service is to be totally free, happy, and master of the universe because then you can be totally giving.

I love seeing Elana now and sharing my ideas with her. I find her to be extremely brilliant and more powerful than ever. She is completely successful and financially independent.

As for Leonard, he has now established a rebirth training center on six hundred acres of land in Sierraville, California, near Lake Tahoe, called Campbell Hot Springs. This beautiful land, containing natural mineral hot springs and an old hotel, was purchased with the help of friends who support the rebirthing process. The Sierraville property was formerly owned by a man who "healed" himself of arthritis in the baths. His symptoms had been the same as those of the birth trauma (paralysis of joints in the hands), although he did not know that at the time. But he had the intuitiveness to stay in the baths long enough so that he spontaneously worked out his birth trauma. He had made an agreement with God that he would save his land for God's work if he could be cured. Many huge corporations tried to buy the precious land, but the man kept his agreement. When he met Leonard and learned about rebirthing he felt that he'd found the perfect people for his land.

I am so glad I didn't quit when the going was rough, because I am just beginning to reap the rewards for the work I have done on myself, and am able to experience the joy of the relationships we established at Theta. On the day cover photos were being shot for this book, Leonard and I stayed in the tub together after the others had gone. Rebirthing each other then was supreme bliss, and I was able to communicate with him on a new level that I have always dreamed about. At one point, I just surrendered to his love from across the tub. Tears shot out of my eyes, then a great white light surrounded me, so intense that Leonard saw it too. I breathed into it and surrendered some more. Leonard put my head on his shoulder and gently continued to rebirth me. Each little breath was like purple fire. It was such a spiritual moment, it was like being in the Bible again.

Recently a small group of us accompanied Leonard on a trip to Europe and to India, where we met a spiritual Master named Abubabaji. Being with this Master was like starting all over, and I spent a lot of my time in Indian hotels, lying in bed and "processing." After the experience has been fully integrated, I want to write about it—and about what it was like to travel with Leonard! At Abubabaji's request, we just broke ground and laid the foundation stone for the first multi-religious temple in Sierraville. The motto is: "Trust in God and respect all religions." This is Abubabaji's purpose, to which we are all now committed.

My other companions now travel all over the country, teaching and rebirthing. We are all financially independent. We try to get together as much as possible because it is so wonderful to be with loving people who have gotten in touch with their own "guruness." We don't have to process each other's cases, we can just experience bliss together. We laugh a lot. It always feels like heaven to me. (After all, heaven is not a place, it is a state of divine bliss.) The disadvantage of being that clear is that people get very "activated," and everything comes up for them after being around you for awhile. If you are a clear rebirther, people's birth trauma will come up for them while they are in your aura. (Many of us have found our bedmates in paralysis after sleeping with us for one night.) So you have to take the position that you are a rebirther and healer twenty-four hours a day. You are never "off duty." But you know, I *never* mind this. I would always be on duty for God. And so would all my companions.

As Rev. Ike says, "You can't lose with the stuff I use!" There is no way to lose when you have handled your birth trauma and become your own guru. Looking back, I find it hard to believe what a mess we once were. Leonard's dream of a multiple guru system has come true.

2 Elana's Story

It's important to realize that Theta Seminars really doesn't exist at all. Rather what does exist is a family of personalities who share in the propagation of a cluster of ideas. I would like to share with you a chronicle of the spiritual awakening of one of those personalities.

I have always prided myself on having an abundance of a quality I call ordinariness. It's the ability to go almost totally unnoticed practically everywhere. I manifested it throughout my childhood, my high school experience proved without a doubt that I was proficient, and in college I excelled at being ordinary. I graduated from Douglass College, New Brunswick, New Jersey in 1966, newly married and slightly pregnant, with a bachelor's degree in zoology. My favorite college classes were animal behavior and genetics. In fact, before I became pregnant and got married, I was considered by many to be a bright young star of molecular genetics. These two details—starting a family life, and my adoration of Watson and Crick (authors of *Under the Double Helix)*—were the principal triggers for the awakening of my conscious evolution.

I embarked on married life, determined and mildly annoyed. My husband was a brilliant young engineering undergraduate at Ohio State University. I was determined that what everyone was naming an irresponsible pregnancy, with disastrous consequences regarding his future as a genius, would turn out OK so I wouldn't have to feel guilty. It was frustrating at the same time that my own career had been put so far onto the back burner that it looked like it had fallen off the stove.

The first three years, we lived in Ohio. It was an easy place to be a good wife and mother, raising a very small person while working parttime as a lab technician at the university hospital. My impatience to be a self only surfaced occasionally in the forms of bitchiness or fits of rage, both unacceptable to me and quickly dismissed as tiredness, overwork or having my period. When my man walked in the door with his master's degree, I felt that my reprieve had happened. I had proven myself a responsible adult and fulfilled my obligation not to ruin his career. When we moved to Palo Alto, California, so that he could study for a Ph.D. at Stanford, I made a secret vow that I would put myself first.

The Bay Area was the perfect place for a young housewife to discover her divinity. In 1969 around San Francisco that's what all the women were doing, married or single—and the men too. Between fall 1969 and June 1973 (when I got fired as "wife"), I actively pursued this list of classes, programs and trainings: Sunday School teacher, two years; Christian philosophy class, two years; Tai Chi and Do-In, weekly for a year; women's consciousness-raising group, bi-monthly for two years; all-day women's meditation retreat once a month for a year; Developing Personal Potential; communication workshop; massage; weekend meditation and encounter retreats; Esalen; ten sessions of Rolfing. I looked at all this as a self-invented Ph.D. program, and never thought of worrying about the cost. I figured it up once, though, and it was about $3,000, not bad compared to three years of college.

During this same period, I meditated daily, often getting up to see the sun rise. I consulted frequently with a brilliant psychic healer, who told me that when I got it straight my life would flow, surrounded by people and filled with accomplishments, money and joy. The pin that burst a hole in my marriage contract was Arica training. At the conclusion of the 40-day intensive training period, my husband cut my Mastercharge card into pieces right before my eyes, terminated our joint checking account, and threw me and my bicycle out of the house.

Except for my guilt about having such a wonderful time, I probably wouldn't have left. As it was, I had a few hundred dollars, a bicycle, two beautiful children living with their father, a miserable previous job experience in the laboratory and a lot of wonderful, mystical, mind-opening experiences. I met a man who took me to an *est* guest seminar and I enrolled for the next available training. Sitting in the Jack Tar Hotel for 60 hours, I "got" that I was actually well-trained, and had something to offer people as a self-improvement "guru." I felt that I possessed, in addition to ordinariness, qualities of kindness, purposefulness, and a childlike sense of fun. In the week following my graduation from *est* I invented the form around which I would sell my newly evolved personality characteristics. The course outlines for two classes emerged.

Miraculously, the local "Y" and recreation department agreed to list my classes in their calendar and a psychiatrist I knew supported me in arranging one for some of his clients. I was launched into the self-improvement business with an average monthly income of under eighty dollars. It was a wonderful time; I assisted regularly at *est,* spent three days a week and every other weekend with my kids, and my confidence as an effective group leader grew even as my savings account dwindled. After about six months, my meditation began to indicate that there was more to be learned about life than I knew. I would begin to look for still another idea, another "guru," something that would synthesize for me all that I had learned of biology, genetics, human psychology, child-rearing, religion, my experience of myself as a group leader, and my lovelife. I signed up for a dream workshop that Lynn Proctor, who had studied at the Jung Institute in Switzerland, was leading at her home.

On Tuesday, March 5, 1974 I had a dream. There was a man, standing in the basement of an abandoned school. He was the teacher I was searching for. I was on the top floor pressing the button for the elevator so I could descend. The elevator seemed to be stuck. I became frantic, rushing about looking for a way to be with him. Then I was in the classroom and he was teaching the class. I wanted the lesson and yet, even there, the trapped frustration was present. The next day I told my dream to Lynn. Her hypothesis was that the dream was about a new teacher, soon to come into my life, who could give me what I had been longing to know. She believed that the trouble I had getting to the room and the feelings I felt with the dream man were a warning from my intuitive nature that I could lose the centered feeling I had so carefully nurtured at the expense of my marriage.

On March 7, 1974, in a huge auditorium filled with people listening to Werner Erhard, I took a seat next to Leonard Orr. He seemed like a friendly person and was handsome enough. I gave him my phone number and Saturday of that same week, he was sitting on a chair on my porch when I walked up with my eldest son's new train set under my arm. We spent the first day of our relationship attaching the parts of the train and fixing the switches and track pieces to the board. The most remarkable thing about him was that he spent an entire day sitting in my son's bedroom, reading instruction sheets about trains. He didn't even know us. I remarked to myself that he was a man who really enjoyed children and their activities as much as I did.

He stayed for supper and, while my children were out playing, asked me, quite pointedly, what books I had been reading. It happened that I was reading the Old Testament book of Exodus. He said that was good. (I thought, "What is this? a quiz?") He asked me to tell him a little of what I understood so that he could straighten out my thinking. ("This guy is a bit presumptuous.") He said that he had taught a class on the Bible once. I had gotten Moses and the folks into the wilderness by then and just about had the Jews up to discovering the Promised Land.

Leonard told me that the reason Moses never reached the Promised Land was that he was a man who saw himself separate from God. The wilderness represented confusion and the Promised Land is self-realization, realizing that you and God are one. "Now there's an idea I never heard before." Immediately I went for the toilet, and while I was sitting there eliminating body wastes I eliminated some mental garbage as well. As I started downstairs again, a wave of energy passed through me. It was as if I had taken a fast-acting drug. I saw myself as a flower, with real roots into the ground—I could really feel them going through both floors of the house and into the earth. There was a sun above, radiating energy into my petals. It all went all the way through. There wasn't any separation between me and the energy flowing and the earth. It was a "rush," waves of energy that made my cells vibrate.

By the time I returned to the dining table, my face was flushed and my whole body was tingling. Leonard laughed and said, "What happened to you?" and hugged me. I struggled to hide myself, my mother's warning that I always wore my heart on my sleeve took hold of my thoughts. I don't remember how I did it, probably one of the kids came in for a drink, but somehow safety was restored. Leonard and I were again in a safe conversation about our pasts and our ventures into the self-improvement business.

We came to an agreement that I would invite a group of my friends to a Sunday afternoon seminar he would lead called "Spiritual Psychology." We set the date for two weeks later. The price was ten dollars. I felt that two weeks wasn't enough time for me—and how *ever* would I talk people into paying ten dollars for an afternoon seminar I hadn't even heard yet? Actually, it was the improbability of succeeding that made it exciting to play. If I was successful, it would be an outrageous miracle. I agreed to supply a minimum of ten paying guests. He agreed to split the profits with me. Very little mathematics was needed to show that I could walk away with a forty dollar profit after a ten dollar printing investment. That meant my income would increase by 50 percent in one month!

My friends in *est,* Quaker meeting, the dream group and my own classes all thought the price was too high, yet they couldn't help noticing my radiant face. On March 24, there sat fourteen of them in a borrowed living room. Theta Seminars was conceived! (My income had nearly doubled in one month!) Leonard's presentation was embarrassingly unprofessional. Not only did he speak so quietly that you could hardly hear, but he also sighed heavily throughout, picked his nose, and cleared his throat loudly. While most of his material seemed well-organized and thought out, it appeared to lack the dramatic impact of the *est* training. Then he started presenting his ideas on the unconscious death urge. Actually, looking back, it would have been much easier for me to pay attention if I hadn't been so involved with wondering what my friends thought of him. As it was, the minute I heard the words "physical immortality" I shut down my hearing completely. I felt betrayed. Here I had invited all my friends, charged them ten dollars, and he was bouncing off-the-wall irrational ideas like that! From deep inside my mind, I remembered that no matter how much I had resented him for intruding into my secret life as a Bible student, he had done it so successfully that my face was transformed forever. Perhaps these friends weren't as critical an audience as I. I looked at them secretly and was struck with their faces. All of them looked to be profoundly confused, yet they too were radiating, glowing with life. They were perplexed and happy at the same time! At the end of the afternoon, he asked how many of our guests would be willing to come back and half of them raised their hands.

Later, we picked a Sunday in April to present a seminar called "Self-Analysis." He suggested that if everyone who raised their hands brought two friends I could double the number of people at the seminar by doing half as much work myself. $7 + 14 = 21$. I would find only seven new faces and pocket $140. Was I willing to have an attendance goal of 28? "Yes, but let me tell you what a crummy public speaker I think you are first." As I finished enlightening him about how he could clean up his presentation he asked me to get out a clean sheet of paper. He told me that I was too hard on myself, my self-esteem was low and I should work with these affirmations for the next week: (1) I like myself, I am a lovable person; (2) I am highly pleasing to myself; (3) I am highly pleasing to myself in the presence of other people; (4) I am highly pleasing to others and others are highly pleasing to me.

It was obvious from the start that I would enjoy writing these affirmations daily in a notebook. I had never said such nice things about myself. I could immediately see that using them until those thoughts became habit would change my critical perceptions of others as well. That he seemed unwilling to acknowledge the validity of any of my criticism of his presentation made my doubts all the more persistent. It was impossible for me to accept that all that I had perceived was inappropriate information based on my own low self-image. If so, then I was really a little shit. If my perceptions were even partially accurate then they had value and he was using my psychology as an excuse to dismiss me. Emotionally, I felt dismissed, blamed, and unjustly accused. There were two ideas developing in my mind: the first was that he had something of great value to share, and the second, that I would have to master it thoroughly in order to have a conversation with him where it was impossible for him to use my ignorance of my own nature to his advantage. I had invented a game in which I could multiple my income, transform my personality, and improve the quality of my own material, and the goal was to be able to have a conversation with Leonard in which we participated as equals.

I used all the skill I had in organizing those first few seminars. I had learned, through *est,* some skills in talking to people on the phone so that they would want to hear me. Leonard had given me a list of metaphysical books to read. I was already leading a class on how to set and realize personal goals. I was inspired by my desire to be self-employed and my certainty that, as a woman, I would never be offered a very big salary. In this business it was clear right from the start that I invented my income. In April, thirty-three people came to our Self-Analysis Seminar. (I doubled my monthly income in one day.) As I remember, we had two seminars in May with about thirty-five at each, and in June we signed in 140 for "Money." In the month of June, Leonard went to work fulltime for *est.* Werner asked him to not give outside seminars while he was with them. We had by then, an active mailing list of over two hundred. He called me to tell me he wasn't giving seminars and why didn't I give them myself.

From the first time Leonard gave me those affirmations until my first seminar incorporating my interpretation of his meta-physical/psychological philosophy, my ideas about motherhood and my ideas about men and sex had been bounced around on a stormy sea of confusion. Each time Leonard visited me, my brain would come up again for review, my beliefs were questioned, evaluated, scrutinized, tossed out and replaced with a new set of affirmations which I would diligently write. The affirmations served as a curative for a shattered mind, writing them soothed me, and the immediate results they produced restored my self-confidence.

Leonard's idea about kids was that they should pretty much do what they wanted to, and their parents should too. The kids telepathically pick up instructions from their folks and love to follow them. The only conclusion a parent can draw from that simple philosophy on an everyday level is that if your kid won't eat his spinach it's because your mother forced you to and you've secretly hated it ever since. If your kid interrupts you by crying while you're having coffee with a friend, it's because you believe that mothers never get time off. Your kid sucks his thumb when *you* feel insecure. As divine beings, children neither need "proper" food nor "proper" sleep; they have enough self-direction to accomplish these things easily. If as a parent you enforce bedtime or certain foods, it's to get the kid out of the way or get even with your parents and has nothing to do with his needs. Rivalry between children is created by the parents belief in scarcity (there's not enough love to go around) coupled with the ancient idea that children should be rewarded with love for being good. Obviously if there is nothing a child can do to be "bad" then they are loved all the time. A child who is loved all the time has nothing to resent or rebel against and therefore is a cooperative person who respects his parent.

I spent hours everyday those four months, watching my children, watching myself relate to them, and writing affirmations to correct what I had observed. When their behavior upset me uncontrollably, I would scream affirmations at them, about how I had a right to get my own way all the time, or something. Quite often, yelling these affirmations triggered a vivid childhood memory and I would find myself totally absorbed in a primal experience. Instead of screaming at the kids, I was actually screaming at one of my parents. When that happened it was wonderful, because I was crying for myself and not to make my kids be different.

In those moments I was asserting myself in a real way for the first time in my life. I didn't care anymore what the kids did. They could be hungry, crying, tired, fighting, I didn't care. I was holding out for number one—myself. In those moments, the kids behaved in the most remarkable way. They watched me. They waited for me. They offered to help me. They asked me why I was crying. They coached me by saying, "Why would your mother say that to you, Mama?" The older one, who was seven, one day offered to take the younger one, who was three, out to dinner on his bike. On his bike to the Jack-In-The-Box, five blocks away, on a major street, riding double. I didn't care, "Sure, go, and bring me back a hamburger. I'm not leaving this floor." I sobbed my heart out the whole time they were gone. Not for them, though, for me. They came home a half-hour later safe, fed and with dinner for me. That's when I got it, just how divine they are. It was so clear that if I was being real with myself, even if it was really miserable, they were real with themselves, which was warm, loving, generous and cooperative.

In under four months, my relationship with my kids was totally transformed through my own experience with them and my application of simple truth. I felt confident and enthusiastic about sharing my realizations with other parents. So, when Leonard suggested I lead a seminar, "Parent-Child Relationships" was a natural. The seminar was a big success and still is one of my favorites. The information is so simple and so valuable that parents always love it. Soon, it will be organized into a book so that all parents can get happy about their job, while letting the kids relax too.

The seed of Leonard's seminar on loving relationships is that you can only have one to the extent that you love yourself. In interacting with a member of the opposite sex, that person tends to become, in the mind, the opposite-sexed parent. In ignorance, we relate to them out of the same disapproval we felt as children. Combining disapproval with our traditional guilts about sex and fidelity, it's no surprise that so many marriages are doomed from the beginning.

I was able to see clearly the ways that my husband had resembled my father in relating to me. I saw how afraid I was of being hurt by him. I had always blamed him for my unwed pregnancy. I had resented how he came through it looking like the gentleman doing the right thing while I was the calculating whore. You could safely say I was a man-hater. Leonard's most valuable contribution to my sex life and ability to have loving relationships with men was that he made me so angry and frustrated that I wanted to kill him several times. He's a fairly athletic person, so that no matter how many blows I intended, I was never able to hurt him. I got angry because he was so right that even if he was wrong, he was right. My father was like that too; the scary thing about my father was that if I was right and he thought I was wrong, I was the one with the bruised behind. I hated men because I was afraid of them, and they scared me the most in a conversation where they wanted to be right—especially if I was wrong. Leonard and I had many conversations like that during those early months. He provided a safe environment for me to feel my anger, sorrow and fear, and resolve many of my feelings.

It is a good thing that my connection to infinite intelligence is infinite. Leonard couldn't really crack my case with men, because he was one, so I limped along with it as best I could using affirmations whenever I would. My connection to God was enough that, blinded by fear as I was, I started to see how powerful the mind of a woman is when she decides to get her way with men. It was through these unsuccessful attempts to relate with Leonard that my other relationships underwent radical improvement. I repeatedly hit rock bottom with him and, once you decide it can't get worse, it always gets better. The most powerful conclusion I came to was to treat my lovers the same way that I treated my kids—to use those relationships to my spiritual advantage and hold out for being myself when the affirmations didn't work (when I didn't get my way). I went through several men being hostile, bitchy, aloof or frigid whenever I felt like it, yet gradually I began to notice that they didn't beat me up, even if I was "bad."

I developed the same genuine compassion for men that I had for the kids and the more angry I got, the less angry I was. I started to see that most men were afraid of women, afraid the woman would leave, or afraid she would dominate them. The "male-chauvinist pig" is a scared boy, using his strength and dominating personality to control women by convincing them that they are weak and helpless. The women get sold to the extent that they get resentful, bitchy, and spiritually so lazy they fail to notice how much power they have. In ignorance, women misuse power, becoming hostile or sullen. As a woman begins to experience her power she uses it to give men freedom, to raise their self-esteem so that they feel loved by her and safe in that. She gains security by giving it away to a man. No man will leave a woman who freely loves him. As I began to master this lesson in myself, several men came into my life, willing to be loving friends, lovers or whatever. I got smart enough to accept their love rather than mistrust it. It was the beginning of the most wonderful relationships I had ever had with men and the end of a short, lonely career as a "man-hater." Receiving affection from loving men was the healing balm for my hurt-little-girl memories. It was discovering my female power that gave me the strength to be open to their attention.

Throughout those four months, Leonard and I were frequently each other's house guests. We had great times playing together at the beaches and in the parks around San Francisco. We had spent a week together in Monterey playing on the sand dunes. When we were outdoors together we were always very happy and loved each other very much. It was when we were indoors that one or both of us would begin acting strange. I did it by being bitchy, he did it by getting sullen in the bathtub or carrying on in a strange way in the night.

He would lie in the bathtub for hours yelling things like, "You can't do that to me, you bastard," or "I hate you, you bitch." When I would go in to see what was the matter he would glower from under the water. I would be inwardly terrified yet he would emerge from the bathroom laughing, in a great mood and never reveal a word of what he had been doing. He would cough and splutter in the night. Sometimes he would get up and hang upside down over a chair. If I asked him, he would mumble something incomprehensible about his birth trauma. One day he said to me, "Look, you are going to have to start working out your birth trauma too, or I won't be able to stand being around you." I shivered at the threat of his leaving me.

I really did love being with him, so I did what he suggested, which was to take a long hot bath with my head bent back so that me ears and eyes were covered with water. Within ten minutes, I was overwhelmed with the most utter terror, anger and confusion I had experienced. I had seen clearly the "picture" of a doctor's face, and waves of negative emotions rapidly followed. I began to shout, and he came in to rescue me. I told him what was happening and he laughed and said, "See? maybe I'm not so weird." Throughout the following weeks, I added hot baths to my training program which already included extensive reading and affirmations. The affirmations really paid off in the hot tub therapy. Everytime I did those baths I would be screaming, crying or overwhelmed with a sense of hopelessness until a beautiful, life-affirming thought would enter my consciousness. I would catch onto this idea like a life raft and my body and mind would begin to incorporate the peace the idea represented.

With more and more baths, frenzied though they were, my Christian upbringing began to make sense. I read New Testament stories throughout this period, discovering that Jesus talked about the kind of all-pervading love I experienced each time an affirmation rescued me from my fears in the tub. Perfect love really does cast out fear. Perfect love is loving yourself without any conditions—loving yourself even when you are hating parents, God, doctors, and/or yourself. The strongest love/hate emotions I had known accompanied the fear that erupted in my bathtub. Not only did my self-understanding increase from these baths, but my ability to understand others increased to such an extent that people were calling me telepathic.

I could separate the bombardment of sensory information that was coming to me into two categories: emotional reactions that were originating with me from my past conditioning, and emotional signals originating with others, manifesting as signals in my body. We are always picking up emotional signals from others, but usually we don't recognize it. Other people thought I was telepathic because I could put words to these body signals, describing them as the thoughts or emotions that had previously produced sensation in me. What I said would be what they had been thinking or feeling. Over the year I had developed the ability to heal unpleasant body symptoms successfully by designing the appropriate affirmations. Having the ability to accurately verbalize other peoples' thoughts gave me a lot of confidence as a seminar leader.

The second seminar I led, in July 1974, was on loving relationships. It was a success because of my new understandings about men, the telepathic ability I had awakened in myself from rebirthing—and because Leonard had led a seminar on that subject once in Oakland and I had my notes!

In August, things started moving faster. Leonard retired from *est,* led a couple of seminars in Palo Alto, bought a house in San Francisco, announced the beginning of the first one-year seminar class, and we took fifteen of our faithful to a former nudist camp in the hills south of San Francisco for a week. The camp where we held the retreat had a 6-foot diameter outdoor Japanese hot tub. The fifteen people had been to enough seminars to know about the birth trauma and had heard Leonard talk about some of his experiences working through his own. They were eager subjects for our first experience with what we were then naming a "baptism" and later changed to "rebirthing." It was timely that Frederick LeBoyer's first article in this country on "Birth Without Violence" had come out in a popular women's magazine that week.

I volunteered to be the guinea pig. I read the article aloud, then went into the tub with a snorkel. I floated face down, breathing through the snorkel. At first, I experienced quiet, darkness, peacefulness; intruding thoughts were quickly whisked away with an affirmation, a change of posture or a deep breath and blowing exhale. It was a real surprise to me when I found myself flying out of the tub, sobbing, crawling to find somebody, to find the reassurance of some skin. Fifteen people sat around that tub and not one of them could move. They were frozen in confusion. I found a pair of legs and although they were so tense they felt like wood, it was a great relief. I don't know how long I was lying there sobbing, but finally I felt a pair of gentle firm hands—Leonard's. Then more hands, gentle hands and trembling hands, rough hands, soothing hands and frightening hands, all mixed up. I couldn't talk, but I could hear people talking to me and about me. Parts of my body were in great pain. People were moving me, straightening my body out. That was nice. It was wonderful when someone would touch me gently and lovingly in a relaxed calm way. Leonard was saying affirmations to me.

Afterwards when I was lying on my bed I composed a beautiful song which was in itself an affirmation. Both the tune and the words came to me effortlessly. I was peaceful and relaxed, more than I had ever been. I remember, coming out of that room and looking across at the mountains, how clearly I could see each tree. I made a vow that I would never touch someone in a rough, awkward way and that I would be very careful not to be rebirthed by someone who would go into shock. Still, the rebirth was a singularly profound experience. It was similar to what I had read, and always envied, of the mystical experiences of Jesus, John, and many yogis. This first week of rebirthings was delicious. The hot summer sunshine, the hot tub and the adjacent unheated swimming pool were equal contributors with the rebirth process itself in seducing us out of our inhibitions about nudity, and emotional and physical expressiveness. We were cavorting about, playing volleyball, swimming, crying, hiking, singing, sexing, telling jokes, and taking communion. Some of us would be naked while others were fully clothed, and every stage in between. Nobody noticed. It was ordinary, whatever it was you were doing. Just plain folk, immersed in life without noticing themselves.

As the rebirthings continued, Leonard and I found that we were doing it together. *It* was a subtle breathing. We would both sigh at the same time, intuitively noticing that the person under the water was experiencing *something*. Leonard was more accurate than I at verbalizing what it was. For me, I was fascinated that three people were sharing something without talking or touching, and that we knew we were sharing it. The one under water would invariably relax (you could tell by watching the back muscles) as we sighed with them. I began to notice the sensations in my own body rising and falling with my "water-brother." As the week went by, I expressed to myself the emotional states of the rebirthee, and usually I was accurate. Frankly, if you are watching a rebirth and you aren't "tuned in" at this emotional level, it's mercilessly boring. One of our major problems was getting our friends to stick with it. To start each rebirthing, it took perhaps an hour to get everyone out of the kitchen! I did my first solo rebirth that week; one girl consented to give Leonard a break and trust me to be her guide.

Back in San Francisco, a Japanese tub was under construction in the basement of Leonard's new mansion. He had hired a couple of òffice people and the one-year class was beginning. In two weeks the operation had shifted from the Palo Alto area to San Francisco and I didn't even know it. At first I was offended and angry that my nice business which was operating so successfully from my dining room (I had managed to be reunited with my children for several months and was having a very carefree life and making plenty of cash without leaving my home) appeared to be scuttled. I was considering quitting the game when Leonard called and offered me the job of rebirther. Being involved in rebirthing was irresistible. It was so close, intimate, spiritual, educational and fun. It looked impossible to move the boys to San Francisco. The house was located on a busy street in a rough neighborhood. The local school was reportedly awful. The other prospective tenants had voted against children. Rebirthing would be difficult enough to master without the children's interruptions. I appealed daily to the infinite intelligence of life itself to bring the situation to a harmonious conclusion so we all got what we wanted. In less than two weeks, my "ex" begged to raise the boys, sobbing out how he had missed them through the nine months they had been with me. He wanted them back. I said, "Yes," and called Leonard.

The nine months, October 1974 through June 1975, that I was a resident in the San Francisco Theta House, could certainly be called the gestation period of my spiritual understandings. I learned rebirthing by doing, during that period, over four hundred rebirthings. I led one or two seminars a week and would frequently walk into my evening seminar with my hair damp from the rebirthing just completed. Not only was I earning money, I was getting comfortable with varieties of people and my ability to awaken them spiritually.

My understanding of "mother" shifted from principal caretaker of children to person who has and loves children. I visited my children a couple afternoons a week and occasionally invited them to San Francisco for the weekend. It wasn't at all like being a mother. I peeled off layers of guilt, regret and that feeling that no-one-can-take-care-of-my-children-like-I-can until all that was left was friendship, and camaraderie.

I had three close friends while I lived in San Francisco. I shared my three-room suite with a young man who loved to wrestle and play the noisy games I instigated to blow off the psychological steam that rebirthing brought to the surface of my consciousness. The daughter of a longstanding California friend moved into that suite for awhile. Not only was she a calm, competent assistant in the rebirth room, but she was a loving confidante and companion. I could share my "secret" life with its visions, dreams and meditations. She was so telepathic that on several occasions she walked into my room and asked if I had called her. Each time, it was perfectly appropriate for her to be with me. I would begin to tell her the dream or meditation that was happening for me and, in sharing, the meaning would become apparent to both of us at once.

Fred Sharpe looked like a wild crazy man. He plays the piano like an angel, is a slightly sadistic lover, and a very spiritual person. Invariable, if I felt sad, lonely or confused, he would appear at the door of our house. He was happy to play piano for me or meditate with me or make love to me. He could soothe me or scare me with equal facility and switch from one role to the other at a moment's notice. He composed a magnificent accompaniment to the melody which came to me after my first rebirth. He played it so beautifully and uninhibitedly that I actually sang it in public, at the Consciousness Celebrations at Theta.

My belief in the probability of physical immortality crystallized during my stay at the San Francisco Theta House. Two incidents stand out as pivotal in orienting myself toward living forever. Leonard had gone to Los Angeles and returned trailing the contents of his L.A. apartment. He had a seminar on physical immortality scheduled for that Sunday afternoon, and he called to say he would be at least an hour late and could I start the seminar for him. I gulped and agreed to do it. I glanced through a manuscript he had written and had a brief meditation—a fervent prayer, really. It was a good thing I didn't have time to wonder if physical immortality made sense to me yet. I started the seminar in the spirit of "the show must go on." At the end of fifteen minutes, I knew I was doing OK. It was easier than I thought. The ideas flowed simply and logically, the audience was receptive. The more I talked the easier it was. Just talking about immortality was making me feel more at ease and alive. I was glad to turn the seminar over to Leonard when he appeared two and one-half hours later. At the same time it was proven to my soul that physical immortality is a "natural."

On January of 1975, Theta got a letter from Infinite Survival, a group of immortalists based in Sacramento and headed by Chadd Everone. Leonard was invited to a weekend meeting at Lake Tahoe to map out with them the future of immortality. He wasn't able to get away until Sunday so I went as the Theta representative. On Friday, each of the fifteen present at the meeting shared, as an introduction, the history of their personal involvement in physical immortality. It was clear from the start that the group would polarize around the medical approach and the metaphysical approach. There was rich information, freely given to enlighten me about recent scientific advances in the cure of aging. Chadd Everone's passion for gerontology and human genetics is documented in recent studies published in authoritative scientific journals. His collection of articles, slides, flow diagrams and photographs offer "scientific credibility" to the conquest of mortality. My old genetics training rekindled, I set about proving to myself, until no doubt remained, scientifically or metaphysically (the synthesis is close at hand), that physical immortality is within the realm of human potential. I'm not going to give you the details here, of how I synthesized metaphysics and science for myself. If you really want to know, come to a seminar on unraveling the birth-death cycle sometime. Soon, you may get to read it in a book. The important thing for this story is that I did it, and that once that bridge was made, I felt ready to put myself and my ideas out there in the world.

It's very inventive, how God deals with time. Ideas can stew around in a mind for months and, once crystallized, the universe presses from every corner to assure that a good idea gets to be public domain. Leonard was invited to speak at the national Rolfer's convention in July. As a result, Rolfers over the country were begging for rebirthings in their hometowns. The house-committee-to-take-over-the-local-rebirth-business was pressuring me to live elsewhere with increased intensity.

My marriage had heaved its final sigh in divorce with a joint custody agreement which gave him the children for the school year.

Leonard wanted me to consider traveling throughout the east coast. My bags were already packed.

I went to Boston and New York City on my first trip Back East. Creating a business in a community from a nucleus of one or two interested people is very exciting because it demands the very best you have. It's rewarding because you know you're the only one doing it and you immediately see the results of your own efforts. Doing the nearly impossible was how I started with Theta anyway. Little miracles are stimulating fun.

Boston was first. Three people came to my first seminar there. By the time I left for New York ten days later, thirty had been rebirthed. Leonard had laid good groundwork in New York. My seminars were full and he had found a beautiful sunken tub in the spacious bathroom of an innovative New York architect for the rebirthings. My schedule was completely booked.

It was one of those storybook romances, our eyes met across a steamy bathroom strewn with naked bodies, kleenex and nose-plugs. He kept coming into the bathroom to putter around getting his toothbrush or something. He pretended not to notice I was there. I noticed him though and kept asking myself why I was so sure this person, who was almost old enough to be "Pop," who had a very nice girlfriend already, was "Prince Charming."

I waited an hour for him to appear for the lunch meeting I arranged. He engaged with himself in some boring monologue throughout lunch. My faith in romance was steadfast and I left New York convinced the long wait for the Prince would soon be over. By the time I returned to New York, his girlfriend had jilted him. He met me at the airport, I moved into his apartment before we had our first "date." Doesn't that seem a little brash? When you are immortal, you do things like that. You just forge ahead because you just know. Anyway, anyone who loans out his bathroom to let eight people lie around in it every day for nearly a week from 10 A.M. until after midnight has to be immortal, too, to have the patience to withstand all that breathing.

For the past year I have traveled east on alternate months. Now there are One-Year Seminars in Boston, New York, Amherst, Tampa, and Washington, D.C. When in New York, I am always the guest of my wonderful architect friend. He has turned out to be the exciting Immortal I was looking for. I have everything I ever wanted. My children love me and are happy with their father. The boys and I will be together in Florida for Christmas . . . and they all lived happily ever after. . . ever after . . . ever after. You can expect that sort of ending to a story about one person's unabashed surrender to living.

PART II

Basic Principles

How to Use This Book
As a Clearing Process

A clearing process helps you to uncover, isolate and identify those areas in your consciousness that are unresolved so that you can begin to unravel them. I have written most of the rest of this book in a little different writing style from the anecdotal approach of the first chapters. The balance of the book consists of the pure wisdom of Leonard's seminars, and I chose to present it in a straightforward manner so that you can use it as a clearing process as you read. You can be right there in the seminar while you read, and notice what goes on with your body. If your body gets any uncomfortable reaction on a certain line or paragraph, you can mark an X in the book as a reminder that you got "activated" or "plugged in" or upset at that point. Also notice where you "fall asleep," "go unconscious," get angry, start invalidating everything or feel like throwing the book. You will then be aware that there might be something you want to process yourself on. This method will enable you to grow faster since you will know what areas require assistance.

Actually, as you understand and practice these concepts, you will reach a point where you never again need the help of a guru, counselor or therapist. You will be your own guru. Of course, you are your own guru already, but some of us forget that. I had "forgotten" myself for thirty years. Then I met Werner Erhard and Leonard Orr. And then I met me.

I don't mean to say you should not go to a counselor for assistance if you need it. I did, especially if my depression was hanging around. I never tried to "do it all myself, forever." In fact, that is why we have spiritual teachers. We should not fail to take advantage of them. But, if you "go for" the ideas in this book, you will get to the point (especially after the breathing release) where you no longer need a teacher, because you will be so "connected" to Infinite Being that all answers are easily available to you and you will understand and feel that.

Important

One of the main reasons for writing this book was to make rebirthing simple and easy for you. One of the best ways to do that is to give you a philosophnical framework that will help you better understand it. With this knowledge you will have less fear and less drama to contend with than we did when we began.

Reading the following chapter, "The Truth About Psychology," before the chapter on "Rebirthing" will not only assist you greatly to understand rebirthing but it will also provide you with the keys to enlightenment that you can use forever in all areas of your life.

What is contained in the following chapters is surely the greatest gift that I could ever give you. I feel very privileged to have been the one who, with Leonard's guidance, wrote it down. I am more than delighted to share it with you.

It was because of this information and because of rebirthing that I was able to create the LRT and fulfill my greatest mission in my own way. It is my hope that you will become as passionately interested in rebirthing as I have and will likewise be able to fulfill all your dreams and aspirations.

3 The Truth About Psychology

This chapter is divided into two parts:
The first is the spiritual or truth part
The second part is the psychological part.

Our purpose is to get everyone spiritually enlightened. And enlightenment is *certain knowledge of the absolute truth.* "Absolute truth" is that one and only truth that is true throughout all time and space for everyone. And what is *the* absolute truth? The absolute truth is: *The thinker is creative with his thoughts.* The only way you could prove that this is not the absolute truth is by thought or by thinking it is not, thereby proving the axiom. For example, if you say, "No, that is not the absolute truth! The absolute truth is that everyone dies!" that is a thought you have. That is a thought you create which only proves again thought is creative.

The thinker exists between your thoughts whether you are thinking or not. You could use different words to describe the thinker, like Being, Spirit, Space or God, but don't confuse the thinker with the subconscious. The subconscious means "under conscious" and is made up of thoughts you have had before and is created by thought. The thinker is beyond all thought. It is beyond thought in that is controls thought and creates thought. If you think the word *carpet,* the next thought you come up with could be anything, any thought in all of Infinite Intelligence. Infinite Intelligence represents all possible thoughts in the universe, all the possible thoughts that have ever been thought, plus all the ones that have not yet been thought. Your thinker is the ultimate guru. The ultimate guru is you; your guru can teach you anything you can imagine and a lot of things that you have not yet imagined.

Your thoughts always produce results!! So, are you thinking positive thoughts or negative thoughts? Your positive thoughts produce positive results for you, and your negative thoughts produce negative results. *It is as simple as that.* In order to get positive results in your life all the time, you have to convert your negative thoughts into positive thoughts. You can also change your feelings in this same way, since feelings are just structures of thought. Once you understand and accept this, it is irresistible. Just persist with the positive thought until it dissolves the negative thought. Remember, *thought always produces effects.* "As a man thinketh, so is he." Being spiritual means affirming the positive in the face of the negative. Peace is having harmony of your thoughts. If positive thinking doesn't produce results try negative thinking. Some people think negative about positive thinking and it works for them. If you say positive thinking does not work, it won't. If you say your affirmations don't work, they won't.

The thinker causes everything to be, or to happen, with thought. "Thought is creative" is absolutely true because there is nothing that exists that was not created by thought. "In the beginning was the Word, and the Word was with God, and the Word was God." And there was not anything made that was made without the Word. The "Word" is the symbol for thought. So, in the beginning was thought. The beginning was *created* by thought. You have to think up the concept of a beginning before you can have a beginning.

The effects of thought are eternal until they are *un*thought. Therefore, something once thought continues to produce the result, even when you aren't thinking it. The effects of your thoughts go on whether you are thinking them or not.

How do you handle those unconscious thoughts that are producing effects you don't want? You use a technique called *af-*

firmations to bring those unconscious thoughts to the consciousness where they can be dealt with more readily.

Your mind is the sum total of your thoughts. Your personal combination of thoughts make you different from others. Getting to know someone is getting to know the thoughts he holds habitually in his mind. Scientists tell us we have 50,000 thoughts a day, making each of us a highly complex individual, so you can be forever entertained by simply studying your thoughts. Through studying your thoughts, understanding how you control your thoughts and how your thoughts create reality, you can become *enlightened*.

If you are already enlightened, you can dissolve all darkness. If you are enlightened, your thinking will be clear. As long as you think you are *not* enlightened, you will *never* clear up your thinking. So there is a lot of practical value in thinking you are enlightened; then you will have a universe that works for you exactly the way you want it to. Your thoughts can create absolutely anything you desire. Think about what you desire. When something comes up that you don't want, change it.

The principle of the *Great Affirmation* is that God always says, "Yes." If you say, "I am poor," He will say, "Yes, boss." If you says, "I am sick," you will get the same result. Since *you* are God, you always get what you want. It is important to let your mind know what you desire. If you think you are enlightened, you are as long as you think so. If you think you are not enlightened, you aren't. Your thought is the only power in the universe that makes the difference! What practical value is there in thinking you are not enlightened? Give it up.

There is all kinds of practical value in thinking that you are enlightened, and that practical value must be realized in every corner of your consciousness to be free of hypocrisy.

Christian Symbols of Truth

The truth has been expressed in various sets of symbols. One of the most common to us is Christianity. In Christianity there is the

Holy Trinity: The Father, the Son, and the Holy Spirit or Holy Ghost.

The Father is the Thinker.

The Son is the product of the Father, that which the Father generates, his thoughts. So the Sons of the Father are the thoughts of the Father. If you believe in the Son, this means you believe in your own thoughts, that your thoughts are creative. If you believe that thought is creative, then you can save yourself from anything. The Son will make you free.

The Holy Spirit or the *Holy Ghost* is your personal reality, including the external world—the word *holy* means to "set apart." In the New Testament, the Holy Spirit is called the *comforter*. If you left for work in the morning, and when you came back your house had disappeared, that would be a very discomforting universe. If we didn't have the Holy Spirit, then as soon as you stopped thinking something, it would disappear. You could have only one reality at a time; it would not be possible to have an evolving universe without the concept of the Holy Spirit—setting the spirit apart and having it stay there. For instance, a chair is spirit set apart for the purpose of being a chair, your body is spirit set apart for the purpose of being a body, the earth is spirit set apart for the purpose of being the earth. So then the Holy Ghost is Reality. Remember those in the Bible that were filled with the Holy Spirit were always the ones who could produce physical changes? They were the ones who were filled with the Holy Spirit.

Scientific Truth

The other set of symbols is the scientific method. Science is based on the scientific method, which has four steps.

1. Propose a *theory*.

2. Design an *experiment* to test that theory.

3. Keep testing the theory—this is *verification*.

4. Test it many times so that you can believe it. When it always turns out the same way you can call it a *law*.

However, who determines how many times is enough? No scientist has actually tested most of these laws. But they believe them. For them it is superstition then. A perfect example is pure water—H_2O. Most people think that H_2O is the chemical formula for pure water. Leonard did an experiment in high school which relied on pure water and it didn't come out right. His teacher said, "Well, the water might not have had been pure to begin with, and even if it was pure, your instruments might have contained traces of other chemicals, but if the instruments weren't contaminated and the water was pure, our classroom measuring devices aren't precise enough to determine the exact purity of water anyway. If you want to assure yourself that you have pure water you must make it in a laboratory." Leonard then wondered the following. If the only way you can get pure water is in a lab, then how come it is a law of *nature?* If pure water doesn't exist in nature, then how can it be *natural* law? He tried a similar experiment in college. His professor told him, "It didn't come out right because there are other elements present; there is H_3O (heavy water) present everywhere, and you can never be certain that you have a pure compound of H_2O" in the real world.

If experiments don't turn out right, they invalidate the theory. If thought is creative, then the scientist is creating laws and the experiments will work; as long as the scientist has certainty about what he is going to produce, then he produces it.

The point is that all science is created by scientists, because they are thinkers. And since you are a thinker, that makes you a scientist. Your scientific laws are as valid as any other scientist's. There aren't any laws that you can't have authority over and that aren't subject to your personal choice.

Your present choice has to agree or change your past choices, however. Your conscious mind must agree with your subconscious if you desire good results. If your subconscious has a different law than your conscious, then your subconscious will make you look like a fool until it is changed. But all subconscious laws can be changed by insight after insight, and the patient use of autosuggestion.

Psychological Truth

1. If your thoughts created your universe, what were the thoughts that created your personal reality? To discover this, you use the *Analysis Principle.*

2. If your thoughts create your universe, how do you change your thoughts when you want to change your universe? The answer is to use the *Suggestion Principle.*

3. If your thoughts create your universe, then what kind of thoughts should you have? The answer is found in using the *Goals Principle.*

You created your universe by thinking. You have had millions and millions of thoughts and every one continues to produce an effect forever until it becomes unthought. The thoughts aligned and organized themselves into a body of knowledge. We can call this an attitude or structure of thought. These structures of thought are held together by a system called *emotional logic.*

All the thoughts you have had are competing for your attention in your consciousness. When one of your negative structures moves over your consciousness, then you perceive the universe through that negative structure of thought. And once you start seeing things negatively, another negative structure comes in, then yet another negative structure comes in. Things start looking so black and so bad that you finally say, "No matter what happens to me, it couldn't be any worse than what has already happened" ... and that is a positive thought! This positive structure comes in and dominates your consciousness, and then things start looking rosy. Another positive structure starts coming in and things look rosier still. Pretty soon your whole consciousness is dominated by all these positive structures, and then you say: "Things are so good, it couldn't be better—it is too good to last." And that is a negative thought and down you go! We call these *mood swings.* You can keep yourself in a perpetual high by unraveling any one of these negative structures as it enters your consciousness.

Thousands of people have certain structures that relate or

organize themselves into superstructures which we call *personal laws* or *dominant consciousness factors*. A dominant consciousness factor controls more of your thinking than any other factor. If you can isolate these personal laws, then you have dynamite in your hands.

There are several consciousness factors that cause unhappiness. Leonard calls these the "Five Biggies." They are:

1. The Birth Trauma
2. The Parental Disapproval Syndrome
3. Specific Negatives
4. The Unconscious Death Urge
5. Other Lifetimes

The **Birth Trauma** is your introduction to the world. It is the beginning of the "The universe is against me" syndrome. There are preverbal thoughts and preverbal intelligence. Your thinking begins before you are able to verbalize those thoughts; in other words, even before you were born. Therefore, when you were born you were able to make sophisticated conclusions about that traumatic event. Most people enter the world from the womb. The womb is a comfortable place where all physiological needs are supplied. When we are pulled from this ideal environment, we experience a considerable amount of pain and discomfort. Some people whose birth pains were very pronounced literally live out their lives apologizing for their existence. Probably 90 percent of our fear originated with the birth trauma. Some of the generalizations we might have made at birth are:

"Being out of the womb is unpleasant."
"I can't trust people."
"If this is what it is like, I don't know if I want to be here."
"People are out to get me."
"I can't get enough (air, love, etc.)."

The birth trauma is one of the reasons most people don't like to get up in the morning. The bed simulates the womb experience. In the process of awakening, the memory of birth pains are stimulated to near consciousness. These near memories trigger the fear that you will have to reexperience being born again. Warm baths and showers also simulate womb experience. Some people even choose the hospital as a substitute for the womb or Heaven. Even something like smoking can symbolize being back in the womb and trying to get the comfort of having the lungs full as they were in the womb.

Impatience, hostility, and susceptibility to illness and accidents can sometimes be traced back to the birth trauma. Many people feel either too hot or too cold and never experience lasting physical comfort during their entire lifetime because of an unpleasant birth experience. We view the traditional theological description of heaven as a symbolic description of the womb; what people are really after when they seek Heaven is to get back into the womb. People want to go back into the womb because it hasn't been very pleasant since they came out—and it is unpleasant because of the negative decisions they made at birth, which produce negative results. The rebirth experience was created to enable you to go back and dissolve all that.

The **Parental Disapproval Syndrome** is another major cause of fear and negative programming. The syndrome develops as a result of your parents' experiencing disapproval from their parents and their resentment of that disapproval. But they were not able to get even verbally or physically, so their true feelings were suppressed. They didn't receive enough love and affection and found their parents difficult to please. So they spent the rest of their lives trying to get even with their parents or trying to please them to win their love. They constantly had to perform and conform according to their parents' instructions in a futile attempt to win their love. This is later transferred to employers, authority figures, and "society." They found little satisfaction until they had children (you). Then *they* had a captive child who was defenseless against parental hostilities and often coerced into giving them affection when the parents desire it.

To sum it up, parents take out their hostility toward their parents on their children (you). The spirit of the child is broken. Then you, as a child, have to suppress your true feelings until you have children and you take out your anger on yours—it goes on from generation to generation.

The fact is, you were a divine being when you came out of the womb. Your parents began to disapprove of you and you resented it. But you couldn't resist them or get even because you didn't have a big enough vocabulary or a big enough body. The only way you could get even was to do what they disapproved of, which caused more disapproval. So you kept the disapproval syndrome going until you decided you could not win. Eventually you gave up and surrendered your loyalty to your divine nature and decided to follow instructions. So you followed instructions for the rest of your life. And when you got old enough to move out of the house, your parents (after they had invalidated your creativity, initiative, and natural wisdom) kicked you out and said, "Now is the time to succeed." Then you went out and looked for somebody to give you instructions. That is the reason most people find employers and why people find mates. Hopefully, when you get married you will finally have found somebody who knows how to give you instructions, somebody who will solve all your problems, make all your decisions and plan your life for you. And, they don't do it! Your mate doesn't do it because he or she is expecting the same of you.

Behind that desire to have you plan their life for them, mates will express their hostility toward you. *"Falling in love" is the hope that you have finally found a parental substitute.* If you suppress your hostility successfully enough, then you will have a successful relationship. If you suppress your hostilities long enough in the relationship, then the relationship may last long enough to end in marriage. If you continue to suppress your hostility long enough, then your marriage might last long enough to have children. Guess what happens then? You get even with the bastards. You get even with your parents by taking it out on your kids. (It is obvious that people inherit at least a portion of the subconscious minds of their parents as well as their bodies. In fact, financial and marital relationships usually follow the parents' behavior so exactly that it almost seems mechanical.) The ultimate knowledge is self-knowledge and the ultimate freedom is internal freedom.

There are several vehicles by which the parental disapproval syndrome is transmitted. Three of the most popular are bedtime, mealtime and toilet training. You came out of the womb with "divine" energy and you probably didn't need to sleep a whole lot. But your parents taught you that you do need to sleep a whole lot. Sleep is related to the birth trauma and to being in the womb. When you came out of the womb and all hell broke loose, you learned that the world outside the womb was a hostile place. You have gone through the rest of your life protecting yourself from a hostile world during your waking hours. After running around all day protecting yourself, you experience enough tension so that you get tired and you want to go to bed—you have reached the point of not being able to cope, which develops as an addiction. You want some rest from the world, so you go back into the womb/bedroom. You turn off the lights to make it dark, as it was in the womb. You crawl under the covers, which simulate the pressure of the walls of the womb and raise your body temperature. Then you go into a state of preverbal-like consciousness called *sleep*. So by going to bed you have recreated the womb experience. If you stay in bed long enough, your bed becomes a hostile place. It is hostile because your parents disapprove of your staying in bed too long, and they will come after you with sticks.

There is a lot of unpleasantness connected with bed; it is no wonder that some people have difficulty having fun in bed. It can be an unpleasant place, just as the bedroom is uncomfortable because children also get punished by being sent to their rooms. They go there and feel unloved. So it turns out later that those people can screw on Main Street and get off on sex in the back of the car, but in bed, no way! There is just too much tension and too much going on in the bedroom. It is better to make love on the dining room table, if the dining room table is a pleasant place. However, for most people, the dining room table was where they got all the bad news. Your parents criticized you for playing with your food and not cleaning your plate. Eating can make you nervous forever after.

Mealtime is the time when most kids get the bad news. That's when you learn if you don't clean up your plate you are not loved. So whenever people feel anxiety they go "clean up" a plate.

Then there is toilet training. Now if you had unpleasant toilet training and you go to the bathroom five or six times a day (and you "plug into" those unpleasant emotions every time you go to the bathroom), then it is no wonder you have difficulty ever being happy and experiencing bliss. Problems of constipation, diarrhea, etc., are probably all ultimately connected to your toilet training. I had one client whose mother was so obsessed with toilet training that he developed an anal fixation, became homosexual and could only get off sexually with anal intercourse. He took enemas constantly.

Being aware of parental disapproval is very valuable, because when you are disapproving you are just "running out" your parent, or replaying your parents' tape. The idea is to express your hostility toward your parents and get it out. This will ultimately enable you to love them more. Otherwise, when your parents die, you experience failure. You never "got even" and now you are never going to get their love either. You feel disappointment for having suppressed your true nature and for not having gained their approval.

Specific Negatives are your favorite negative thoughts that you beat yourself with regularly. Here are some favorites: "I am not good enough," "I can't do it myself," "I am a born loser," "Nothing works the way I want it to," "I'll never have enough money," "People don't like me," "Life is a rip-off," etc. It is important to pass judgment on every thought and invert all the negatives into positives. The ultimate specific negative is that death is inevitable. This leads to the fourth consciousness factor.

The **Unconscious Death Urge** is the belief that death is inevitable. The habit people have of affirming the power of death causes not only death, but also many illnesses and states of weakness leading to death. Scientists now suspect that the reason death has been so popular for so many centuries is simply because no one ever questioned it. Some scientists are now declaring that man can banish death altogether from his experience. In reaching this conclusion they are merely reaffirming what the spiritual masters have been trying to teach us for thousands of years: There is an alternative to physical death and that is physical immortality. (Or, not dropping your body.) The alternative to aging is youthing. For a complete understanding of how this can work, turn to the chapter on Physical Immortality in this book.

All information from **Other Lifetimes** would be available to each of us, were it not for the birth trauma. Most people "went unconscious" at birth and experienced pain, drugs and hypnosis, which caused them to lose awareness of their other lifetimes. From an unconscious state, when we begin to look or explore our past lives, we usually are looking to expand the ego. This life is so rough and lousy that we are hoping our former lives were better. The purpose and value of knowing about your past lives is obvious: You don't have to repeat the traumas and negative patterns you experienced in them. Another reason would be to get in touch once again with talents that you had before.

Conscious examination of other lifetimes can give you understanding of some of your deep-seated patterns and can enable you to make connections regarding your unconscious death urge. It will become clear to you that all the ways you died in previous lifetimes have not worked. You can therefore consciously avoid repeating those ways in your present life. You can see how, after having died many times, every way imaginable, you can finally give up dying and create a body that will stay around forever.

As Bobbie Birdsall says, however, "If you had other lifetimes that were more significant, you would be in those." The main point is that exploring past lives is fine, if that is what you want to do. If you get value out of it for yourself, great!

The Suggestion Principle

The suggestion principle is based on the idea that you can improve or control the quality of your thoughts. It is based on taking responsibility for the quality of your thoughts. It is also based on dissolving the lies that you have bought from other people throughout your life.

The Thinker has some fundamental qualities and those are the qualities of life itself: harmony, wisdom, power, love, eternality and infinity. These are the substantive qualities, and the substantive qualities are omnipotent. When you resist or when you have negative thoughts about the essential qualities of life—harmony, wisdom, power, love—you are resisting omnipotent force. If you cling to these negative thoughts long enough, they will cause excruciating pain. *Pain is the effort required to cling to a negative thought.*

Every individual who enjoys living or who wants to live and wants to be happy has to purify his mind of negations of the substantive qualities of life. It is totally impossible to have peace, permanent peace, and bliss, effortless bliss, until you weed out of your mind the negative directions you are giving yourself.

One of the substantive qualities is power. Since you are alive, you are power. As long as you are saying, "I am weak," however, you are resisting the truth. As long as you resist the truth, it will cause you pain. And the more pain you experience, the weaker you will feel. If you progressively identify with weakness, then ultimately weakness will lead you to nonexistence. Power will go on but you won't; you will have used your power to destroy yourself.

Another example: Fear is just a mild form of pain. There is one ultimate fear, the fear that "the pain won't go away." As long as you are clinging to that idea, the effort of keeping the idea will cause more pain. Then you will be convinced that it will never go away.

The suggestion principle uses various techniques to concentrate or control your thinking. The techniques to control your thinking are:

1. Pure thinking, meditation (pass judgment on every thought)

2. Talking (a catharsis: the more precisely you verbalize the negative, the easier it is to erase the thought)

3. Reading (select good, pure literature)
4. Writing (most powerful because it involves all the senses)
5. Listening (collect good ideas from seminars and cassettes)

Go through life collecting good ideas and thinking about them as much as possible. Then when you are writing, you are writing positive thoughts, and when you are talking you are expressing positive thoughts. Actually you are expressing affirmations, either positive or negative, all the time you are talking. The affirmations given in this book are examples of good thoughts that you can collect and work with repetitiously in order to get positive results.

We are beginning to produce more and more tapes which are very helpful, easy ways to program your mind positively. The reason people get bored with good ideas tapes is that it takes a lot of effort to hang on to the destructive thoughts that are being confronted while listening to the tape. Boredom is the effort involved in suppressing something.

The Affirmations Technique

An affirmation is a positive thought that you choose to immerse in your consciousness to produce a desired result. You do it repetitiously until the desired result is manifested. Your mind will create whatever you want it to if you give it a chance.

There are various ways to use affirmations. Probably the simplest and most effective way that we have found is to write each affirmation ten or twenty times on a sheet of paper, leaving a space on the right margin for "responses" of the mind or "emotional reactions" to it. The affirmation is written on the left side of the page; jot down on the right side of the page whatever thoughts, considerations, beliefs, fears or emotions may come into your mind. Keep writing the affirmation and observe how the responses on the right side change. A powerful affirmation will bring up all the negative thoughts and feelings stored deep in your consciousness and you will have the opportunity to discover what is standing between you and your goal.

The repetitive use of the affirmation will simultaneously make its impression on your mind and erase the old thought pattern, producing permanent desirable changes in your life! Thoughts produce results, and since realizations can very soon be discovered with this approach, the results are often startling. Be sure that you are willing to take on the added responsibilities, the new adventures and challenges that will manifest as a result of your breaking the old mold.

The subconscious mind can be impressed like a piece of clay. It is helpful and more powerful to experience the *feeling* and the *visualization* of the affirmation as you say or write it. Remember, affirmations are very powerful and need to be carefully worded.

At the end of this chapter is s sample list of affirmations on self-esteem. Appropriate affirmations are also given at the end of each chapter pertaining to the subject.

Making Affirmations Work For You

1. Work with one or more every day. The best times are just before sleeping, before starting the day and especially whenever you feel depressed or discouraged.

2. Write each affirmation ten to twenty times.

3. Say or write each affirmation in the first, second, the third person:
   I, Sondra, am increasing my willingness to be loved.
   You, Sondra, are increasing your willingness to be loved.
   She, Sondra, is increasing her willingness to be loved.
   Always remember to put your own name in the affirmation and keep it in the present tense. Writing in the second and third person is also very important since your conditioning from others came to you in this manner.

4. Continue working with the affirmations daily until they become totally integrated into your consciousness. You will know this when your mind responds positively and you

begin to experience the intended results. You will then be experiencing mastery over your goals.

5. Saying the affirmations aloud works if you repeat them regularly on schedule; for instance, five minutes in the morning, five minutes at noon, and five minutes at night for about seven days.

6. Record your affirmations on cassette tapes and play them back whenever you can. You can switch on the tape recorder when you are driving or when you go to bed. Record each about ten times (slowly) so you have time to think about them.

7. It is also effective to look in the mirror and say them to yourself outloud. Keep saying them until you are always able to see yourself with a relaxed happy expression. Keep saying them until you eliminate all facial tension and grimaces.

8. Another method is to sit across from a friend, each of you in a straight-back chair with your hands on your thighs and knees barely touching each other. Say the affirmation to your friend until you are comfortable doing it. Then have him say it to you in the second person. Your partner can observe your body language carefully: if you squirm, fidget, or are unclear, you do not pass. He should not let you go on to a new affirmation until you say the first one very clearly without contradictory body reactions and upsets. Also he should continue to say it back to you in second person until you can receive it well without grief or embarrassment.

If you are writing affirmations, it is a good idea to stop using the response column after a week or so in order to avoid indulging the negatives that come up. You could switch to a tape recording. It is also effective to type affirmations. However, an advantage in doing them longhand is that you can observe your handwriting changes as anger, or other emotions, come up.

As you read over the sample affirmations, note which ones have the greatest emotional reaction or "charge" for you and mark them. The ones that you have the most resistance to are the ones you should definitely do. Work on no more than three per week and then let go of them and let them sink into your subconscious.

You have probably heard friends repeat over and over again some complaint or negative statement. They were making negative affirmations which will produce negative results for them. However, their statements can produce negative imprints on *your* subconscious, too. It is always beneficial to be around positive people.

Watch your own words (which are just verbalized thoughts). Catch your own negative statements. As the Bible says, "Thou shalt be ensnared by the words of thy mouth." What you say is what you get; what you think is what you get. The Day of Judgment comes when you reap the results of your thoughts.

Self-Esteem Affirmations

1. I _____ like myself. I am a lovable person.
2. I _____ am highly pleasing to myself.
3. I _____ am now highly pleasing to myself in the presence of other people.
4. I _____ am highly pleasing to others and others are highly pleasing to me.
5. I _____ am a self-determined person, and I allow others the same right.
6. I _____ have the right to say NO to people without losing their love.
7. Other people have the right to say no to me without hurting me.
8. I _____ like myself, therefore I like others.
9. I _____ like myself, therefore others like me.
10. I _____ like others, therefore others like me.
11. I _____ like others, therefore others like themselves.

12. The more I like myself, the more others like themselves.
13. I _____ am attractive and lovable and the more I acknowledge that, the more true it becomes.
14. My defense mechanisms are no longer necessary because I am a wonderful person.
15. I _____ deserve credit for my success and accomplishments whether it was difficult or not.
16. I _____ am now a worthwhile woman (man) even if I am _____.
17. I _____ can satisfy myself in the presence of anyone.
18. I _____ am now willing to give up my act of _____.
19. The more I enjoy being alone, the more I enjoy being with others.
20. I _____ am loved and appreciated whether I am with someone or not.
21. I _____ am a winner whether I like it or not.
22. Fulfilling my own selfish pleasure makes me a responsible person.

Goals Principle

Make a list of one hundred things you would like to do—everything that you have ever wanted to do. Then make a list of one hundred personality traits or qualities that you would like to combine, talents you would like to have. Then make a list of one hundred possessions that you would like to have. From the total of three hundred goals, pick out one and concentrate on it, think about it, and make up affirmations for it. Write it on a card and carry the card with you and think about it every time you have a minute. Just concentrate on that one goal until you attain it. Then, after it materializes, pick another one and think about it until it materializes. And then pick another one and think about it until it materializes. When you have conceptualized and materialized several different goals, you will have a success consciousness, which means all you will have to do is think about something and it will start to materialize itself!

When you have a success consciousness and have materialized ten or twenty goals, read over your list and you will notice that twenty-five or fifty of them have materialized and you didn't even work on them!

4 The Rebirth Experience

Introduction

The purpose of rebirthing is to remember and re-experience one's birth; to relive physiologically, psychologically, and spiritually the moment of one's first breath and release the trauma of it. The process begins the transformation of the subconscious impression of birth from one of primal pain to one of pleasure. The effects on life are immediate. Negative energy patterns held in the mind and body start to dissolve. "Youthing" replaces aging and life becomes more fun. It is learning how to fill the physical body with divine energy on a practical daily basis.

Rebirthing is about 99 percent pleasurable. Some people call it fun! The one percent of rebirthing that is not enjoyable is due to your unwillingness to give up your misery. All discomfort in conjunction with rebirthing comes from holding on to negativity, misery or pain. The perfect divine energy that moves in your mind and body during rebirthing is your own pure life force cleaning the dirt from your soul and body. This energy frees you from all harm by making you aware of how you hurt yourself everyday (if you do) so that you can stop.

This perfect energy that flows into your body as a tingling sensation is God's healing power; the tingling or vibrating sensation is the cleansing action of God's love on the psychic "dirt" in your

71

body and aura. God's energy does enter your body from the center of your cells. Rebirthing is an experience of opening your breath so that a special flow of spiritual energy washes your mind and body with a divine bath. This spiritual bath has many sensations. Some people feel fear or sadness or pain in the process of being freed from their unpleasantness, misery and sickness. But most people let go of their fear right from the beginning and love rebirthing.

It is impossible adequately to describe rebirthing. People usually tell us that "It is far more wonderful than anything you said." Obviously, God's energy can heal all human problems. Rebirthing is the science of letting in God's energy, wisdom, and love. Rebirthing has been called an intuitive science, but all words are helpless and crude in the middle of the experience.

Rebirthing is a spiritual gift! In itself it is perfect and harmless. However, when you apply perfect spiritual energy to a mind that has been conditioned to know fear and pain and all kinds of negative things, then the conditioning is exposed and you can let go of it. You can let go of human misery to be a free and natural person. Your human personality can be filled with serenity, joy, health and spiritual wisdom. Rebirthing actually delivers more of these things than we can possibly promise. The reality of them is far more glorious than the words. We have not been able to say anything too good about rebirthing because rebirthing, as we experience it, is God's power in your human form. Only your own personal divine goodness can feel it and know it. It has been called "a biological experience of religion."

To get the most out of a rebirthing experience, it is valuable to do it with a loving person who has been trained in the wisdom of how these spiritual energies work. It is also necessary to raise the quality of your thoughts as you experience rebirthing, so that your mind is in harmony with your perfect divine energy. The more efficiently you raise your thoughts, the faster healings take place.

You may notice that there are apparent contradictions, confusions, and unclarity in this book. That is because it is the story of real people struggling to incorporate perfect divine energy into words and into their human forms. If we waited until we could say everything right, it might take forever and you might never benefit.

Therefore, it is for your benefit that we are publishing it now. We give you our stories with love in the hope that our truthfulness about our imperfections will cause you to laugh and to love us. We believe that our mistakes will save you from committing the same ones. We believe that our honesty will inspire yours.

We don't know if rebirthing is a religious experience or not. If rebirthing is religious, then breathing is religious. Rebirthers, from the beginning, were self-employed. Each rebirther is an independent business person. The secular professional mode seemed to be the best form to use in the beginning because it is free and honest. However, as more and more church people and academic people experience rebirthing it will be seen more and more in those environments.

We feel that there will always be a place for the high quality work of well-trained professionals.

The Birth Trauma

At the moment of birth, you formed impressions about the world which you have carried all your life; these impressions control you from a subconscious level. Many of them are negative:

Life is a struggle.
The universe is a hostile place.
The universe is against me.
I can't get what I need.
People hurt me.
There must be something wrong with me.
Life is painful.
Love is dangerous.
I am not wanted.
I can't get enough love.

Your impressions are negative because your parents and others who cared for you didn't know what you needed when you were born, and gave you a lot of things you didn't need: Lights that were too bright for your sensitive eyes, sounds that were too harsh for your ears, and touches of hands and fabrics too rough for your delicate skin. Some of you, despite the fact that your spines had been curled up for several months, were jerked upside down by your heels and beaten, which produced excruciating pain. Breathing became associated with pain and your breathing has been too shallow ever since.

But the physical pain is nothing compared to the psychic pain of birth. Nature provided that as a newborn you could receive oxygen through the umbilical cord while learning to breathe in the atmosphere (which was a totally new experience after having been in water), but the custom has been to cut the cord immediately, throwing you into a panic where you felt you were surely going to die right at birth.

Another significant psychic pain occurred when you were snatched away from your mother and stuck in a little box in the nursery. Most people never recover from this mishandling of the separation of mother and child. For nine months you knew nothing but the inside of your mother's womb. It was warm and comfortable until it got too small for you. What you needed was to be shown that the world outside is a far more interesting place, with a lot more possibilities than the womb, and that it could be just as comfortable, safe, and pleasurable as the place you had been. However, since your leaving that place was so traumatic, you have probably spent your entire life trying to get back there, never noticing or experiencing the full extent of the possibilities out here.

Fortunately, there are now some changes being made in the birth process. Frederic LeBoyer, a French obstetrician, delivers babies in dim light, with few sounds. He places each child on the mother's stomach, holding him gently, and waiting for the child to learn to breath on his own. He cuts the umbilical cord only after it stops pulsating, and holds the child gently in a tub of warm water to show that there are comfortable and pleasurable experiences available outside the womb. The warm water immersion re-creates the feelings of being in the womb. In the tub of water the muscles relax, the baby experiments with movement, a smile may appear. Several doctors in this country have adopted this method, and they say that "LeBoyer babies" are more relaxed, cry little or not at all, and seem to expect love and pleasure from their universe. They are brighter, less afraid, and almost never sick.

At the same time as Dr. LeBoyer was developing his process in France, Leonard Orr in California was discovering a way of helping a person at any age to get in touch with his birth trauma and remove it from consciousness.

* * * * * *

Sitting in a sauna one day, Leonard noticed a sign that said: "It is recommended that you stay in the sauna no more than fifteen minutes." Typically, he decided to stay there longer and find out why there was a suggested limit. His experiment ended when he crawled from the sauna and almost passed out. Later he came to believe that he had gotten "plugged in" to the memory of life in the womb, and the memory had blocked out his consciousness. About this time he noticed that he was having trouble getting out of the bathtub; he would get all kinds of insights into infancy if he stayed in the bath for a very long time. He started to do this regularly. He even learned to sleep in the tub. And so Leonard began the long process of unraveling his birth trauma, which led to his creation of the rebirthing technique, in his own bathtub.

* * * * * *

The process Leonard created is very simple and yet extremely powerful. In the beginning, all rebirths were done in a hot tub. The rebirthee entered the tub with a snorkel and noseplug and floated face down while the rebirther and the assistant gently held him in place. The water proved a powerful stimulus in triggering the experience of being in the womb and being forced out of it. In fact, as the process evolved, it became clear that going in the water for the first rebirth was so powerful that it was too scary for some people. To avoid overwhelming them, Leonard devised the dry rebirth, which is primarily used today. He had noticed that it is the breathing and relaxing in the presence of a rebirther that is crucial to the success of the rebirth, and not the water, as he'd thought originally. The process works best when a person is dry-rebirthed until he has a breathing release, and then moves into wet rebirths.

Rebirthing occurs when people feel they are in an environment safe enough to re-experience their birth. Being in the presence of a rebirther—someone who has already worked out his or her own birth trauma—gives the rebirthee the certainty that "I will come out OK." The message is communicated, telepathically and emotionally, to the subconscious mind of the rebirthee; in addition, the rebirther will verbally encourage him by a gentle reminder that he survived his own birth the first time, and can do it again.

The rebirthing experience varies from person to person. As each discovers his negative conditioning, the rebirther assists in the process of rewriting the script by using affirmations. These are written to contradict specifically the negative decisions the person made at birth. So we create the view that:

The universe and my body exist for my physical and mental pleasure.
I can get all the love I deserve.
I am glad I was born; I have the right to be here.
I am safe, protected by Infinite Intelligence and Infinite Love.

Needless to say, when a person begins to adopt this view of the world his life changes drastically. So, for all of you who have ever dreamed of being reborn and starting life all over again, you can now make it possible!

In addition to healing the damage done by the birth trauma to the individual consciousness, it has been found that rebirthing repairs the damage done to the breathing mechanism at birth and removes the blocks where the inner and outer breath meet, so that Infinite Energy and Infinite Being always becomes easily available to the human body. Ultimately we may learn that rebirthing is a physical experience of Infinite Being which is not exclusively to do with the birth trauma. We do know from experience that rebirthing merges the inner and outer breath, which creates a bridge between the physical and the spiritual dimensions. This connection unites the human body to the prenatal life energy that built it originally, and thereby rejuvenates the body and frees the individual consciousness, not just from the birth trauma, but any kind of trauma. However, the birth trauma does seem to be the major obstruction to the unity of inner and outer breath.

Any negative thought will inhibit the breath, but the most destructive, inhibiting thoughts are negative ones about the breath itself. Therefore, the negative thoughts you had about life itself while taking your first breath are the most damaging to your breathing mechanism. Reliving your first breath is one of the focal points of rebirthing and is one reason why we continue to call this spiritual, mental, and physical experience *rebirthing*.

After the rebirthing is completed, the merging of inner and outer breath and its rejuvenating effect becomes spontaneous and effortless. That is, breathing fully and freely with the spirit, mind, and body becomes the natural way for the individual consciousness to function. When rebirthing is completed in an individual, and the power of the breath is restored, spiritual enlightenment, the affirmations principle, and other spiritual techniques or philosophies (like Yoga or physical immortality) become all the most important because of the significant personality changes. Rebirthing cuts away human trauma at such a fundamental level that the people who complete it are transformed from working on themselves to playing in the universe. All self-improvement games become recreation and leisure activities which enlighten, rather than serious business. Rebirthing puts fun into self-improvement as well as into life itself.

Here, in outline form, are some of the things a new rebirthee should know.

    I. Basic philosophy: Everyone is divine and has the responsibility to rebirth himself.

A. We are not willing to take responsibility for consequences of anything that happens *but*
B. If *you* are willing to take responsibility, we are willing to
   assist in any way you feel appropriate.
C. Rebirthing yourself is as easy as anything else. Like
   skiing or playing piano, you can do it the easy way or the
   difficult way.
D. So far rebirthing has worked on everyone who has a
   navel. Having a rebirther somehow substitutes for the
   mother- child relationship and provides a quantum leap
   in the quality of the experiences.
E. The easy way is to find somebody who has already
   worked out his or her birth trauma.
F. While mastering the physical manipulations involved,
   you may also pick up psychic certainty from the person
   teaching you.

II. Unique aspects
A. Rebirther: a person who has worked out his or her birth
   trauma and become familiar with divine energy.
B. Rebirthee: a person willing to re-experience the primal
   life force and let go of the birth trauma.

(In the rebirth you are unlearning a negative skill *i.e.*, being tense
all day long.)

The Breathing Release

Rebirthing is merging the inner and outer breath to experience the
fullness of divine energy in the physical body. Re-experiencing
birth is only necessary as long as it is inhibiting the breathing
mechanism; so we have stuck with the term rebirthing and applied
it to physical birth because the basic inhibition on the breathing
mechanism was implanted on the individual consciousness during
the first breath. It is also called rebirthing because in each session
the divine infant is born again in human flesh.

The breathing release is the most important aspect of rebirthing. It is a critical release of all your resistance to life. The breathing release happens when you feel safe enough to re-live the moment of your first breath. It is physiologically, psychologically, and spiritually reliving the moment when you started to breathe for the first time. The breath mechanism is freed and transformed so that, from that moment on, a person knows when his breathing is inhibited and is able to correct it. This experience breaks the power of the birth trauma over the mind and body. A portion of the breathing release probably takes place in all genuine rebirth experiences, but the climax occurs when vibrating energy goes through the throat, usually causing constriction and choking just as on amniotic fluids when you took your first breath. This is the scariest part of rebirthing because the person goes through the first moment of his life when he struggled to breathe while drowning, suffocating and strangling in an attempt to get amniotic fluid out of the breathing passages and air in. That closeness to death must be cleared away before a person is safe. It is getting a person through this moment that is the art and primary role of rebirthing.

The breathing release puts the power of your life-force into your thoughts. Therefore, be careful what you think about when you are breathing! The danger of having the full power of aliveness without the wisdom of awareness is that you may destroy yourself more efficiently. We have noticed, however, that people who are destructive usually don't get rebirthed. If they try, they usually are unable to "let go" until they give up destructive thoughts.

It should be obvious that human beings have more power than they are willing to acknowledge. As a direct result, we commit the ultimate sin: not recognizing that we are God: thinking we are not God originally came to be because Eve failed to recognize God in herself. Original sin is transmitted through birth trauma which invalidates a child's divinity and rebirthing is a scientific method of regeneration.

The breathing release comes easier for people who understand their unconscious death urge and have worked out a philosophy that includes a concept of physical immortality. I had spent fifteen years working out my own unconscious death urge before I met Leonard. That, together with his teachings of physical immortality (which I grasped readily) and my deep trust in him, enabled me to go through most of the breathing release the first time. By then I was aware that I was responsible for my own life and death and that no thing outside myself could kill me. This reduced my fear tremendously. It is scary because, if your umbilical cord was cut before you learned to breathe and you were literally about to strangle to death on your own amniotic fluid, your birth trauma may be the closest thing to physical death that you have ever experienced. Re-experiencing the moment you learned to breathe may be so frightening for you that you may not be willing to do it until you have worked out your death urge. On the other hand, people who achieve the breathing release are able to drop their fear of death, and their connection to their physical body sometimes becomes so pleasurable that physical immortality spontaneously becomes conceivable and desirable. We desire that rebirthing contribute to your aliveness and recommend that you master the section on physical immortality.

Hyperventilation

Hyperventilation is the breathing release in process. Hyperventilation (medically described as breathing so deeply that there is a dramatic loss of carbon dioxide in the blood) is usually treated as a disease. It is actually the cure for subventilation. Subventilation is inhibited breathing, commonly called *normal* breathing. Hyperventilation is impossible for a person who breathes uninhibitedly.

It is important to discuss hyperventilation because many people think that it is something to fear and make the rebirthing experience more difficult for themselves than is necessary. One doctor who was particularly afraid of hyperventilating set the all-time record of five hours for a rebirthing by resisting it all the way through. Several hundred other doctors relaxed and went through it without difficulty.

What is called "hyperventilation syndrome" is a natural part of rebirthing. After rebirthing over ten thousand people, we have evolved a new theory of hyperventilation which is unanimously accepted by medical people who have completed their rebirthing. The new theory is that hyperventilation is a cure for subventilation. The birth trauma inhibits a person's breathing mechanism, causing shallow breathing. When a person breathes normally, fully and freely for the first time, without fear, it automatically produces some changes in the body. After watching ten thousand people successfully make it through a hyperventilation experience, we have concluded that all the person requires is calmness, safety, and encouragement to complete the process. If the person is encouraged to be patient, to breathe naturally and to relax while experiencing his fears, no harmful effects occur. On the other hand, if this natural process is interrupted by either the fear of the participant or the observers, the result seems to be perpetual fear of hyperventilation and its accompanying symptoms.

Our research has made the the old theory obsolete. We are not medical researchers, but we have been told by several doctors that one theory about the cause of hyperventilation is that it is caused by rapid breathing. We have found in all ten thousand cases that the rapid breathing cleared up the hyperventilation syndrome—including tetany and other accompanying characteristics—rather than caused it. We may not have the sophisticated technical machinery that the medical profession has, but since we have cleared up over ten thousand cases of the hyperventilation syndrome with rapid breathing, our theory deserves respect. The theory is that rapid breathing may accompany hyperventilation syndrome, but it is more a cure than a cause.

We have found that if a person has a voluntary rebirthing experience once a week until completion, it produces a feeling of profound health and well-being. After a person has relived the moment of the first breath, then hyperventilation syndrome no longer occurs. A person can breathe as fast and as hard as is physically possible without any undesirable effects. Therefore, our conclusion is that hyperventilation is a natural cure and not an illness.

In our work we learned that breathing fast was not necessary to induce the hyperventilation syndrome; we observed that relaxing in the presence of the rebirther produces the syndrome regardless of the breathing speed. Increasing the breathing speed, as long as the breathing is relaxed, eliminates the elements of the syndrome completely. We apologize to the medical profession if we are doing their work for them, but it was an accidental discovery on our part and we are willing for them to benefit from the research.

In January 1977 Leonard made a report on this to the National Institute of Health. They have since begun investigating these theories and invite him to Washington, D.C. regularly to benefit from his work.

After observing over ten thousand cases, we concluded that although some physiological (chemical) explanations have some value, none of them fit all cases. We concluded that the only common denominator is fear and that all physiological processes seem to be controlled by psychological causes. Leonard defines fear as the effort involved in clinging to a negative thought which negates a substantive quality of Infinite Being. Any anti-life thought can cause what is called tetany in medical terminology. Rebirthees usually call this phenomena cramps, paralysis, or the "creeping crud." The phenomena doesn't occur with rebirthees who relax into the "tingling" energy sensation, who stay with a constant breathing rhythm, and who allow themselves to feel their fears. People who try to stop the energy and protect themselves get paralyzed. The cramps may be repeated for a few rebirthing sessions until the negative emotion can be verbalized and released. Then the individual can permit the tingling and vibrating energy to flow freely and evenly throughout the whole body.

When the energy flows evenly and freely in the body, it heals, balances and grounds the person. The rebirthee feels a profound sense of peace, serenity and physical well-being.

This state seems to be permanent. Individuals who pursue rebirthing to this point report that simple breathing power is a whole new source of health, energy and pleasure.

If the Biblical symbol for breath is fire, then hyperventilation may be the baptism of fire which Jesus talked about. If this is true then it leads to the bizarre conclusion that what is considered by the medical profession to be a disease is a major technique of spiritual enlightenment and cleansing.

The Energy Release

At some point in rebirthing there is a reconnection to Divine Energy and as a result you may experience vibrating and tingling in your body. It starts in different places in different people and, before rebirthing is complete, it usually is felt throughout the whole body. This energy reconnects your body to the universal energy by vibrating out tension which is the manifestation of negative mental mass. Negative mental mass can be permanently dissolved by continuing to breathe in a regular rhythm while your body is vibrating and tingling—experiencing your reconnection to the Divine Energy.

Major Points of the Energy Release

1. Relaxation causes inner and outer breath to merge and the breath opens.
2. When the breath opens, the merging of the inhale with the exhale brings about the experience of Infinite Being on the physical level.
3. This breathing cycle cleanses the mind and body; there isn't necessarily any tingling or vibrating with this cleansing process.
4. If there is resistance or fear, then the body will tingle and vibrate. The vibration is not the energy but resistance to the energy. However, vibration is the cleansing process and should be welcomed. Resistance is negative thought previously impressed on the mind and body. At the completion of a breathing cycle resistance is dissolved and the person is breathing faster and there is no tingling. Understanding this is helpful for people being rebirthed the first time, otherwise they will have no way of knowing that rapid breathing eliminates the tingling. The assumption that

most have is that rapid breathing *causes* the tingling.

5. The truth is that rapid breathing is dissolving and pumping out tension and negative thought from the body and vibrating is incidental to the cleansing process.

6. After the cleansing, Divine Energy is coming in with every breath. There is no sensation, but the increase in vitality and health is evident in the body and one experiences bliss in the mind.

7. The energy release is actually dissolving resistance to Divine Energy.

The energy release in the body is so dramatic that many people are afraid of the vibrating sensations and try to stop them. Since the energy is your own life-force, you should not try to stop it. When you try to stop your own energy moving in your own body, it causes tightness, cramping, or temporary paralysis. Consider what your mind might go through at this point: The body is reconnected to the pleasure it felt when it was in the womb. The last time you experienced that much pleasure it led to your birth and the resulting trauma. Therefore, you believe that something terrible will happen again. This is where the pleasure precedes pain philosophy started; that is, the bliss and pleasure of the womb led to the pain of the birth trauma. So the pleasure being experienced through the vibrations creates a fear of the "inevitable" (which never happens). In experiencing a pleasure for the first time, we concern our minds with how we will eventually have to pay for the enjoyment, to the detriment of the pleasure. Therefore, you might try to suppress the vibrations to reject the sensation of your own life-force. If you try to stop these vibrations, however, a painful conflict will occur and you can paralyze yourself temporarily. *Paralysis is caused by resisting yourself.*

One part of your mind says, "I want to do this," and another part says, "Hold it, maybe I don't want to do this." This conflict results in paralysis in the body. It is the same conflict we had at birth. "I want to get out of the womb" and "I don't want to leave." The fear of irreparable damage is the idea that "If I go out of the womb, I'll never get back in." This fear of irreversible change is the origin of all fear. (This is also the basis for the fear of death.)

The paralysis usually lasts only for about ten or fiteen minutes although the fear is that it will be permanent and that it will cause irreparable damage. When it is over, you might think that the energy caused the paralysis. But it was *not* the energy that caused the paralysis! It is fear and resistance to the energy that caused the paralysis. However, if you believe in your mind that the vibrations, which were actually pleasurable, caused the pain, then you might keep resisting. When you felt pleasure and were afraid something terrible would happen, and something terrible did happen, you might conclude that you were right to try to stop it. You might think that, if you hadn't stopped that energy, something even worse might have happened. So the tendency is to keep resisting, and it gets worse. And each time it gets worse, you probably would conclude you did the right thing. You might want to say to yourself, "If it got worse when I tried to stop it, what would have happened if I hadn't tried to stop it?"

Not everyone goes through this erroneous reasoning process, but the people who do continue to close down and go into fear until the pain becomes excruciating. When it reaches that point, they finally start to let go and follow the instructions of the rebirther. As they breathe more efficiently, the paralysis immediately lessens. However, as the paralysis releases, the vibrating or tingling resumes dramatically. This usually frightens them and they close down again. Some people experience many such cycles until they can relax and breathe at a rhythmical speed. You can avoid all this if you will only let go to the experience of feeling your own life-force in your body.

Rhythmical breathing is pulling on the inhale and relaxing on the exhale in a continuous stream so that the inhale is connected to the exhale. The key is to relax into the tingling.

Rhythmical breathing empties the negative mental mass out of your body and enables you to incorporate the life energy into your body instead. If during the energy release you are willing to trust the instructions of the rebirther, in regard to your breathing, you can move through the energy release with a minimal amount of discomfort. Unfortunately, since the birth trauma is the original source of distrust, you might at this point enter into a period of distrusting of the rebirther and nothing that the rebirther does or says will seem correct. You may continue in the pain and if you are in pain you will blame the rebirther for the pain that you are causing yourself.

A negative thought stored in your body automatically resists the aliveness of Infinite Being. The presence of the rebirther automatically lowers the resistance; the rebirther can help alleviate your pain. Cooperation is the best thing you can do for yourself. Completion is when you become a good rebirthee and do it right.

People who become temporarily paralyzed in rebirthing may be more fortunate than people who don't, because they learn two things: One, as soon as they get in touch with their fear of the symptoms and let go of that fear, the paralysis ceases and their body opens and feels pleasure; they learn that behind all pain and fear is pleasure which is God's love. Two, if they don't get in touch with the fear and verbalize it but relax into the symptoms and keep breathing, the paralysis goes away anyway. So they learn that healing is inevitable whether they understand or not!

Therefore rebirthing is a model for all healing. The elements are as follows: Relax into the symptom so that you can get its message about your mind. Don't be afraid of it. Pain and fear are the effort involved in clinging to a negative thought. Behind all fear and pain is pleasure, which is the physical manifestation of the metaphysical love of God. All pain, all fear and all illness is resisting the pleasure of God's love and wisdom on some level.

Pleasure is natural. All else is unnatural . . . and ultimately self-destructive. If you don't relax into the pain and go through it to the pleasure that is behind it, life will become too much of an effort and you will love death more than life. *Death is loving pain more than you love pleasure.*

For people who don't experience the temporary paralysis, we can only assume they have mastered the pleasure-pain principle previously through some other means or that they may go through it in the future. The few people who are able to go through the rebirth experience without paralysis also have the ability to let go completely. The ability to let go during the energy release is based on trust.

The energy release gives you a new body. You feel connected to your body in a wonderful way—sensually—abundant physical energy and a sense of safety and serenity spreads over you. When the rebirthing experience is complete, this serenity becomes permanent. The primary thing that could interrupt it is the negative mental attitudes of others in your environment.

During rebirthing you need to trust that in the universe there is no natural force that will hurt you. Trust that it is your own mind which creates what happens in your body, and that you can uncreate it. Trust that the vibration is good energy that will heal you and mobilize the tension and negative mental mass, enabling you to breathe it out. Trust that the tingling and vibrating is "God loving you at a cellular level." Trust that the energy sweeping through your body is restoring your primal ability to experience pleasure and serenity. Trust your rebirther who has taken hundreds of people through the experience and every one survived. If you survived your birth, you will survive your rebirth!

Pictures

During rebirthing, possibly even the first time, you can achieve total recall of your birth scene. But you may become so preoccupied with your physical body that you will care very little about memories and pictures. However, the pictures usually become more and more obvious with each subsequent rebirthing session and after you have worked out the physiological stuff, you can sit down quietly at any time and recall events surrounding your birth. In other words, after the trauma has been removed, you will have the tendency to gain full memory of your birth experience and the events surrounding it. I have rebirthed several people who were adopted and had no conscious recall of their natural parents prior to that day. In their rebirth experiences, they were literally able to "see" their natural mothers and fathers and give me incredible details about their lives, which enabled them to understand and forgive the parents for having given them up for adoption. Hundreds of other people have remembered details they were never told. These details were then related to their parents, checked out and confirmed, to the amazement of the parents.

The main reason some people have trouble remembering their birth is the negative mental mass inhibits them from remembering anything before age five or three. A good affirmation to remove this memory block is, "My mind is immersed in Infinite Intelligence which can deliver information to me about my past, present and future." Memory blocks caused by past traumatic experiences are a common subject of psychology. The theory is that painful experiences are blocked from the memory because the person does not want to remember the pain. Our theory is that remembering the experience releases the pain and frees the mind and body; and that the release is not painful, but sometimes intensely pleasurable. The fear of painful memories holds the pain in the mind or body to be experienced as pain or tension. To free your memory you have to get rid of the concept that remembering painful incidents makes the pain worse; and you have to get into the idea that the release is worth the time—and wonderful.

Rebirthing is focused on releasing rather than re-experiencing the trauma. Most people, when taking out their household garbage, don't find it necessary to examine each individual can, bottle, wrapper, and box before discarding it. However, it is a curious phenomenon that those same people, before letting go of any "psychological garbage," will find it necessary to meticulously pick through, sift, taste, touch, smell, analyze, classify, examine, and understand each item in order to make sure they don't throw out anything valuable. Using this analogy, we say that if psychoanalysis and psychotherapy are like diligently picking through your psychological garbage in an attempt to understand it, then rebirthing (in most cases) is like carrying out your garbage in one fell swoop. In the beginning some people find this very disconcerting, because the rebirthing process releases negative mental mass so quickly you don't have time to think about or understand it. After the rebirth, however, most people are so high and feel so good that they could not care less about "understanding" it.

Symptoms

We think of rebirthing as the ultimate healing experience because your breath, together with the quality of your thoughts, can heal anything. We have seen symptoms, from migraine headaches to sore ankles, disappear as a result of rebirthing. Respiratory illnesses, stomach and back pains have disappeared. Frigidity, hemorrhoids, insomnia, diabetes, epilepsy, cancer, arthritis and all kinds of manifestations have been eliminated. These illnesses seem to be caused or prolonged by the birth trauma. People get stuck in birth trauma symptoms and develop medical belief systems about them. Doctors then become mother-substitutes to support an infancy act. In rebirthing, we see people go through physiological changes in ten minutes that other people stay stuck in for years and from which they may die.

On the other hand, rebirthing creates a safe environment in your mind and body for symptoms from the past (example: childhood illnesses and patterns) to act themselves out. It is well to keep in mind that these symptoms are temporary and relatively easy to eliminate with the powerful ally of uninhibited breathing. But if in your mind you are afraid of these symptoms or resent them, you may inhibit your natural healing powers. Some of these symptoms can be bothersome and frightening. It is well to use physicians that you can trust, as well as spiritual and mental healers, to make it easier for you to get out of the traps in your own mind. Rebirthing is not for people who retreat from life in fear, who desire to curl up and die, unless they want to break up this pattern. Rebirthing is for people who are dedicated to aliveness and who desire to live fully, freely and healthily in spirit, mind and body.

It might be helpful to discuss some examples of temporary symptoms that may occur as you work out your birth trauma.

Some people have re-experienced childhood earaches after re-birthing. Some have experienced spontaneous generation of veneral disease symptoms (diaper rash symptoms). If you are in complete agreement with medical belief systems about VD, you may indeed experience irreparable damage. But after watching all kinds of VD symptoms clear up as a result of rebirthing, we believe that VD may be an adult manifestation of dirty diapers and feelings of helplessness from infancy, as well as feelings of frustration from unpleasant toilet training experiences. We have found it to be a valuable working theory. We recommend that you use any medical treatment that works for you, but we have found that the results of medical treatment are temporary if the cause is not dealt with. Failure to reach the cause will get you another opportunity to use spiritual or mental techniques each time the symptoms recur. In the end, mental and spiritual methods have to be used to produce a permanent cure. We don't claim that any cure is permanent, because human beings have the eternal power to re-create any symptoms—even physical immortality can be revoked. The breath is the headwater of your life stream, so healing the breath is the ultimate healing experience. Free and full breathing, plus raising the quality of your thoughts about your body, will eventually clear out all prenatal and postnatal imperfections of your body.

Obviously, the complexities of all the personal case histories that we have worked with would take many volumes to relate and if you labored through them, they still may not help you. There is no substitute for trusting your own intuitive wisdom about your own body and having friends around you that you can trust to add their wisdom to yours.

Rebirthing is a spiritual, mental, and physical model for healing. Essential characteristics of rebirthing can be applied to all symptoms by relaxing into the feelings of the mind and body while maintaining a breathing rhythm and inverting the negative thoughts that are creating the feelings.

Remember, all illnesses are actually cures in progress. Rebirthing can be a roller coaster and for some people can be the opening of Pandora's box. Therefore we recommend rebirthing for hearty people who love life. Some people report that rebirthing produces only highs and enriches their bliss and health. Other people report that subsequent to rebirthing, they experienced their highest highs and lowest lows and then leveled out.

Rebirthing creates a safe environment in the mind and body to become free of all negativity; however processing negativity can be overwhelming at times. For this reason, we recommend that you have a rebirth weekly until you feel safe and whole. We also recommend that you make the whole process of your spiritual growth easy on yourself by participating in a human community with enough spiritual, mental and physical techniques to assist you efficiently and to support you in processing whatever changes you might go through. We also strongly recommend that you return to the philosophy of Physical Immortality regularly until you have mastered it. This philosophy sows in the mind the seed of supreme optimism that makes conquering all difficulties an adventure instead of a tragedy.

Holistic institutions combining spiritual, mental and medical and other techniques are rapidly taking over the healing field. The medical profession has traditionally maintained its monopoly by claiming exclusive license on words like "heal," "cure," "treatment," "therapy," etc. It should be obvious that this exclusive claim is a disservice and dishonor to the value of the medical profession, which claims to exist for the humble service of mankind.

Benefits of Rebirthing

People tell us that rebirthing is the greatest experience they have had since they were born. We constantly hear comments like this one: "Every growth experience I've had promised more than it delivered except rebirthing. Rebirthing delivered a whole lot more than it promised." One thing they are excited about is the natural healing they have experienced in rebirthing. We have observed that many diseases are a result of birth trauma symptoms around which medical belief systems have been built; most diseases are actually cures in process. The disease is the body manifesting thoughts from the mind, so that the mind can be changed. That when the message the body is revealing is understood, the disease sometimes clears up spontaneously. Some of the physical conditions that have cleared up spontaneously through rebirthing are ulcerative colitis, common cold, backaches, poor eyesight, migraines, sinus trouble, throat and ear problems, breathing difficulties, respiratory illnesses, arthritis, epilepsy, dermatitis, acne and psoriasis, and chronic tension in the legs and body.

The purpose of rebirthing is not healing; healing is sometimes a valuable by-product. We take no responsibility for the treatment of any conditions, physical or psychological. We recommend those who have a condition they are concerned about stay in constant communication with their physician. Rebirthing is not a treatment and no claim is made as to its ability to cure symptoms or reverse illnesses.

The purpose of rebirthing is to acquaint people with a dimension of spiritual energy which they may not heretofore have experienced. When people are experiencing this process, they are able to connect their illness or pain with the original negative thought behind it, out of which it was created, and therefore take total responsibility for causing it. Some people are able to completely let go of the condition instantaneously during the rebirth. It literally gets pumped out of the body with the breath. Others let go of it gradually during the weeks following rebirthing by utilizing affirmations and their newly altered way of breathing. It seems that, as the yogis have told us for centuries, the breath is the cleanser of the body. Any person who improves his breathing and upgrades the quality of his thoughts experiences a transformation.

I personally eliminated a physical pain that had persisted for fifteen years. I had tried every possible way to get rid of it, however nothing worked. Two weeks after I began getting rebirthed, I was able to let go of that pain permanently. In addition, I let go of all kinds of psychological problems. Throughout our rebirthing of others, we have seen problems resolved like claustrophobia, insomnia, fear of harm, fear of being trapped in relationships, sexual disorders and fears, misplaced anger, chronic distrust, and general fear and anxiety, to name only a few. Rebirthing does not treat these conditions but seems to provide a spiritual medium whereby they can be understood, dealt with, and released. We want to make it clear however, that the birth trauma is not responsible for everything. In a sense, the birth trauma is highly overrated, even though it is often responsible for terminal illnesses and many common maladies that plague people for life, including crippling of the breathing mechanism which may be the result most damaging to human happiness. When rebirthing clears these things up, the damage done by the birth trauma seems irrelevant. It is amazing that when you have a problem, it predominates and pervades everything; but when it is gone, it is impossible to remember what a burden it was. So the birth trauma pervades everything and dominates us until we are free and then we wonder why we made such a big deal of it. This paradox is a tragedy for gratitude, but a benefit to bliss and accomplishment. It is good to be grateful, but sooner or later we have to go on to the process of living. The first step is to let the birth trauma out of its suppressed prison in the individual's subconscious, second, to do the work of healing its damage to the individual's mind and body. And the third step is to become as unattached to the healing process as to the trauma and go on living a successful life.

There are other general benefits that everyone who completes rebirthing receives. One of the most important is the ability to receive love and have the direct experience of letting it in. During rebirthing, you are physically able to feel the difference between resisting the love and letting it flow in, and touching is not required to get this experience. As a result, people begin to experience more and more bliss in their daily lives without working at it. As a result, the physical body becomes a more pleasurable place to be. When old aches, pains, and tensions are gone forever, even just walking can become orgasmic. Another benefit is the increase in psychic awareness. Rebirthed people have more and more experiences of telepathy and intuitive knowledge, which again makes life more effortless, fun, and interesting.

In addition to a healthier, more relaxed body, people experience a great deal more physical energy and less need to sleep. The energy formerly used to keep the birth trauma suppressed is released and available for other and better things. As a result, re-birthed people become more beautiful. A propensity for youth-fulness occurs as well as a desire for physical immortality. After one has a breathing release, the ability to breathe freely and unin-hibitedly becomes natural. This, of course, leads to less effort while working; and therefore working becomes more like playing, especially when people do the thing they love as a career. (I have noticed that people who complete rebirthing will not tolerate do-ing a job they don't like. Since they know the universe loves them and they can trust it, they have no qualms about quitting a job and starting over in something for which they have a greater affin-ity.) As a result, their prosperity naturally improves. Rebirthing also improves prosperity because people are able to let go of the idea, "There is not enough," which started when the baby, chok-ing on amniotic fluid, hysterically concludes, "There is not enough air." This later gets translated into "There is not enough love," "There is not enough money," etc. If a baby did not get the breast milk he wanted or enough of it, this may have been fur-ther compounded.

Another reason work becomes more fun and results in more prosperity is that creative ability is enhanced by rebirthing. This occurs because your personal connection in Infinite Being and In-telligence is restored through the freeing of the breath. This con-nection to Infinite Intelligence gives you the ability to understand your own patterns, to see the truth about your own hangups, blocks, and negative conditions and thus know more how to clear them up by themselves. One of the more important aspects in this area is getting in touch with your own *personal law*. This is your most dominant negative consciousness factor formed at your birth, upon which most of your self-invalidation was built. It is really the key to working out your negative patterns.

The results of rebirthing are not always rosy. The mood swings of an individual's disposition are sometimes exaggerated. Some people report that after rebirthing they experience their highest highs and lowest lows, which eventually level out into bliss. Some people experience pain and other forms of discomfort which seem to be stimulated by the new internal freedom. Statistically, rebirthing is safer than the public schools. It is usually possible to come out of rebirthing in a perpetual state of health and bliss, but the path may sometimes be rocky. On the whole, however, rebirthing is the fastest and most effective technique to higher consciousness that we have experienced. If people experience their birth in rebirthing, they may go on to re-experience various periods of infancy which are wrought with feelings of helplessness and hopelessness. These periods can last for weeks and are sometimes accompanied by symptoms that will be discussed later. Exercises that are discussed later have a tendency to dissolve the "infancy number" the easy way.

Genuine spiritual experiences may cause either healings or sickness. Causes and cures of specific symptoms already exist in the personality, and the spiritual energy activates and releases the person from these cause-and-effect relationships. Pure aliveness always transcends the wheel of Karma and yields greater personal freedom.

Rebirthing ultimately raises your self-esteem to a very high level. And when that happens, all areas of your life are affected. Relationships with parents and lovers often change drastically for the better. One of the most gratifying experiences I have ever had involved a woman who had been rebirthed several times bringing her mother from Europe to be rebirthed with her. The mother did not speak any English, but it did not matter. The rebirth went perfectly. The daughter cradled her sobbing mother in her arms and the mother got through to the "other side." I couldn't stop weeping for joy during that experience.

Pregnancy, Birth, and Rebirthing

Pregnant women who have been rebirthed have had transformed deliveries. Several who have given birth after being rebirthed have told us they had very simple, fast and problem-free deliveries, their babies noticeably more relaxed and contented because they were not subjected to their mother's own birth trauma during labor. "My baby came out like butter" is a typical comment.

Dr. LeBoyer has said that he delivered approximately 10,000 babies before becoming sensitive. Professional obstetricians are either the easiest or the hardest to rebirth: easiest if they have started opening up to the infants and become sensitive, which brings their birth trauma closer and closer to the surface. If they are more concerned about performance, reputation, or income, however, than they are of the quality of their work, they develop unconscious defense mechanisms in order to maintain emotional control when their birth trauma gets stimulated in the delivery room.

Dr. LeBoyer's personal history makes obvious that the closer an obstetrician gets to understanding and releasing his birth trauma, the more helpful he becomes to mothers and infants. Rebirthing is invaluable to the baby business.

The ideal birth occurs when the whole delivery team and both parents have been rebirthed. Ultimately, rebirthing of parents should be done before pregnancy. Mothers who had one or two children before being rebirthed report miraculous results in subsequent births. A woman in Boston who had two cesarean section births was believed absolutely to require the cesarean section mode by the medical team. As a result of rebirthing however, she had a natural childbirth which was pleasurable to her and the infant. The obstetrician was frustrated because the baby popped out before he could prepare the mother by making the incision.

Rebirthing creates a whole new attitude about childbirth. It tends to break family traditions regarding the number of children and to favor smaller families. This is understandable to rebirthers. The reason, in our opinion, is that birthing becomes less compulsive when you have relived your own. It is no longer a vicarious psychoanalytical experience that doesn't work. When you have relived your own birth trauma, then having a child becomes a rational decision rather than an unconscious parental and cultural program.

Leonard rebirthed Frederick LeBoyer in 1976. They found their relationship mutually profitable. Frederick's rebirth was easier than most and still very meaningful, especially in relation to his breathing release. The observations of several doctors who do

LeBoyer deliveries and who have been rebirthed themselves are that the benefits of the LeBoyer delivery are inhibited somewhat after the child spends several weeks or months with the parents who still have their birth trauma. Leonard rebirthed a French mother whose child was delivered by the LeBoyer method. She reported that she had special telepathic communication with her child a few weeks after birth which was lost, and that her rebirth reestablished that connection and communication.

Rebirthing obstetricians and expectant parents is a priority of ours because it catches the problem at its source, but the problem won't be solved until rebirthing becomes a major practice in our society. Therefore, the training of skilled rebirthers has been Leonard's top priority since he perfected the process in 1976 and developed an adequate training program.

When we rebirth a pregnant mother we do two at once. We have rebirthed pregnant women during every week of pregnancy down to the last week. To do it right takes extra gentleness and patience on the part of the rebirther. The results so far have been 100 percent beneficial to the delivery. The reason, evidently, is that everything that is worked out before the delivery can't be transmitted during it. So the infant and mother are better off doing it in stages rather than all at the point of delivery.

Pregnant women are easier than other people because the whole pregnancy period is a certain kind of rebirth experience. In almost all cases women who had one or more children are easier because childbirth is a rebirthing experience.

It should be obvious to obstetricians or anybody who works or studies the field that the particular type of birth trauma is a family tradition that gets recreated generation after generation in spite of all attempts at preventative measures.

An Obstetrician's Story

I trained as an obstetrician in a conventional Midwestern medical center. Birth for me was a crisis of survival and an interruption of my work schedule. I was tense all the way through labors and deliveries, wondering if something bad was going to happen or if I was going to have to do something drastic.

After completing my residency, I was stationed in Colorado and then Korea as an Army obstetrician. I was already beginning to feel dissatisfied with my work. I dreaded the time when a woman would go into labor. The ordeal, the struggle, the crisis of survival would start again. I felt uncomfortable and distanced from the laboring woman and her partner. It seemed I was supposed to be able to do something that I didn't know how to do. I felt that I should be able to make that labor smooth and easy and the birth effortless and joyful; and it wasn't that way at all.

The birth was the ultimate crisis for everybody. The parents, the nurses, the baby and I would all be in a state or more or less controlled panic. The mother would be screaming in agony or pathetically disconnected from the experience by sedation or anesthesia. The father would be desperately trying to comfort his mate or angrily demanding something be done, or in a withdrawn state of helpless apathy. The nurses and I would be exerting tremendous effort to control our own upset while going through the ritual of plugging this woman into IVs, anesthetics, monitors, sterile preps, sterile drapes, and standard positioning in the stirrups.

And what about the baby? The baby was treated with all the respect and concern that any heart-lung preparation in an animal research lab would get. Every conceivable procedure was done to insure that those lungs would fill with air and that heart would pump good blood through that warm flesh. This important package that I believed would some day be the home of a mind, a soul, and awareness would be quickly separated from the placenta, taken to a table under bright lights, vigorously dried and stimulated, usually by flicking the bottom of its feet, tightly wrapped in a bulky blanket, briefly shown to or held by the mother and father, then whisked off to the nursery where it was weighed, stabbed with a vitamin K shot, its eyes inoculated with a burning silver nitrate solution, a thermometer shoved up its rectum, measurements taken. Then it was left alone for several hours except for a watchful eye from across the room.

About two years ago I saw Dr. LeBoyer on television, along

with his film about the gentle, loving birth. I couldn't handle the idea. It seemed like one of those kooky, fringe intellectual ideas that flash into popularity and quickly fade. Soon after that, prospective parents began asking me for that kind of birth. I didn't want to do it. I was uncomfortable with the idea of adding anything to what was already a struggle. I agreed to do it, though, because I was also uncomfortable about saying no.

The first birth I attended with the lights turned down was reassuring. I got through it more easily than I expected. With the next few births I began to notice that the mood in the delivery room was more calm and serene. The focus of attention was now on the baby and parents instead of being scattered out towards instruments, nurses, doctors, placentas, and unrelated idle talk.

I discovered that there was a person inside of that baby, a conscious, aware being that actually responded to my attention and caring. I was moved. My whole outlook on birth took a 180 degree turn. I looked forward to the joy and excitement of being there when a new person emerged into the world.

Then a friend told me about rebirthing. A couple of weeks later my chance to be rebirthed manifested and I went for it. I now know what bliss is all about. I sailed into the highest high I had ever experienced and it was easy.

Since that time I have been rebirthed several times, and each one has been a profound experience for me. I now have, from my own experience, a feeling of connection with those newborn persons. And I know from my memories of my own birth that that recognition of the person inside the baby is what the baby needs more than anything else. That knowing that he or she is a person and not just a flesh-and-bones-machine allows the baby to go through life with a basic sense of self-esteem.

My experience of birth, since rebirthing, has reached a new level of satisfaction. Having worked through my own birth allows me to be there with the baby without getting plugged into my own birth memories.

I love being there as the new being emerges, watching as the initial upset passes. Soon the eyes open and the baby looks out at the world. An amazing calm settles over the baby and everybody else in the room. The breathing is hesitating at first then more and more regular. It's like the baby is getting accustomed to this new experience of breathing. The baby then starts making sounds like talking. I talk to the baby at the moment of birth. I say, "Hi. Welcome to the world. Everything's OK. You're going to like it here. It's a beautiful world. Your mother and father are here; they are anxious to see you. Welcome to the world."

Phil DuBois, M.D.
Seattle

The Rebirther

All professional rebirthers operate from their own divine authority; that is, the rebirther is able to serve his clients truly and well only if he had recognized his own divinity as it derives from his personal connection with Infinite Being. No one is qualified to appoint rebirthers or to discourage them. We support anyone who produces genuine results, whether or not they have been trained by Theta professionals.

However, the exhilaration of the rebirth experience may occasionally lead an unqualified person to begin doing rebirthings without any clear understanding of the process or ability to deal with the kinds of situations that may arise. Enthusiastic friends may make even an unqualified rebirther successful temporarily. Unqualified rebirthers have developed in the past by being rebirthed and using the process without Leonard's knowledge or consent. Others have attempted to rebirth people after having only partial training. Also, rebirthers have started training other rebirthers, and by the time you have several generations of trainees, it becomes both impractical and impossible to guarantee the quality of everyone who claims to be a rebirther.

There is also a spiritual problem involved. Leonard's position is that no one is qualified to appoint rebirthers or to discourage rebirthers. Only God can judge the qualifications of a rebirther.

All rebirthers are spiritually ordained and they must operate, if they are genuine, from their own divine authority. Therefore, anyone who claims to be appointed or authorized by Leonard is "lying" and not to be trusted because that person doesn't trust himself. However, God sometimes allows some strange people to do his work! The rebirthers we certify are willing to accept their own divine authority and support others who have demonstrated the quality of their work to each other.

The rebirthing profession is a perfect work because if the rebirther does not love God, it doesn't work and if the rebirther doesn't love the rebirthee, the rebirther won't have the patience to do the work. And since the method is invisible, if the rebirther doesn't have love and true power from God, the clients won't pay. So it is impossible to pervert the profession of rebirthing. In other words, the power of rebirthing work is so great that if the rebirther's consciousness is not pure enough, both the rebirther and the rebirthee will be "wiped out" (made ill) by the process itself. In this way God protects misuse of his power ultimately; but the damage that is done can only be cleaned up by a person who is pure and truthful. It has also happened that someone might see the profession of rebirther as a way to make money, gain fame, or go on a power trip. It is reassuring that such people inevitably fail to become established rebirthers. We have seen rebirthers motivated primarily by money get sick very quickly and quit the work. We have seen rebirthers motivated by fame or a power trip get frustrated and quit because their clients called them on their "number." The power and virtue of Divine Energy exposes all fraud.

Nevertheless, we do want you to be aware of the desirable qualifications for a rebirther, so you may confidently select one for yourself. The selection of your rebirther is a very personal task, and in a sense it can be thought of as choosing a compatible loving companion for a journey you will be taking on your own. We are all our own gurus.

In 1976 Leonard conducted a training program on the East Coast which led to the establishment of certification designed to maintain the quality of our work. Because I was unable to attend,

I have asked Kristian Kelly to write the certification story. It is not too long ago that Kristian turned in his scissors and gave up being a well-known hair cutter in order to become a rebirther. It was not long ago that Lynda, his lady, turned in her wings and gave up being a stewardess in order to become a rebirther. They are now one of the top rebirthing teams in the country and are leading rebirth trainings with outstanding results. We are most fortunate to have them with us and you can see them both on the front cover of this book.

The Certification Process

A nine-week training program for rebirthers that took place during the summer of 1976 in Walton, New York culminated in the establishment of a certification process. Leonard designed the process to insure high standards in rebirthing people and to maintain those standards by certifying individuals who have demonstrated their ability and received the unqualified support of all their associates.

"What qualifies a person to be a rebirther?" Leonard asked the sixty people who were present at Walton that summer. Each one responded by stating what he or she felt characterized a rebirther. All comments were recorded and the session continued until there was complete agreement in the room that all points had been covered completely. It was apparent that the response was a direct reflection of the individual's intuitive connection to Infinite Intelligence and Infinite Being. The following is a complete list of the qualifications rebirthers must meet in order to be certified.

Prerequisites for Rebirth
International Rebirthers

1. The ability to produce results with your clients:
   (a) completion
   (b) release of body tension
   (c) release of conditions related to birth trauma

2. Completion of oneself—having unraveled the substance of ones own birth-death cycle and parental disapproval syndrome
3. The ability to function without outside approval from one's clients and colleagues for one's well-being and feeling of success
4. The ability to conduct successful rebirth seminars
5. The ability to create successful affirmations
6. The ability to function successfully in a spiritual community
7. The ability to function effortlessly and pleasurably in the physical universe
8. Motivation other than money
9. The ability to remain confident and competent while experiencing helplessness and/or weakness of oneself
10. Confidence in one's intuition
11. Respecting and valuing the divinity of oneself, clients and colleagues
12. Have completed, or presently be a member of, a one-year seminar (subject to negotiation)
13. The willingness to continue evolving and training as a rebirther
14. Functioning successfully, including financially, as a rebirther for a period of three months
15. The willingness to support other qualified Rebirth International rebirthers and members of Rebirth International
16. The ability and willingness to create support groups for your clients in all areas in which you work
17. Obtaining the written agreement of ten Rebirth International rebirthers
18. Having attended a rebirther training for one or more weeks at a training center

Certification of those present began by Leonard's asking another question: "Who qualified as a rebirther according to the prerequisites we have just established?" Everyone was standing. The room hummed with skepticism, trepidation and humor. Of the sixty people present, thirty-five sat down and twenty-five remained standing. Beginning with a premise that all are equal in all ways, the thinning of the ranks was rapid and breathtaking.

What was then demonstrated was the most efficient, honest and thorough system of individual selection imaginable, leaving little doubt as to the results produced. As individuals were confronted with reservations about their abilities to rebirth people, they sat down, while the rest of the group continued standing. Those sitting down could still voice objections about anyone left standing.

The room took on a heightened consciousness and a deep feeling of spirituality. Intuition pervaded the assembly. The selection continued until there were only five mildly frightened bodies standing. These five vertical bodies had met the agreed-upon qualifications, and they had the unqualified support of everyone in the room. Those seated had demonstrated and accepted that they themselves did not have enough certainty on one or more points of qualification to remain standing.

Out of twenty-five people who started this process, five people were certified.

The result of this session was the guidelines and format for subsequent rebirther certification which, of course, we are always upgrading. Success in being certified was the direct result of a candidate's personal certainty on meeting the stated requirements. The Walton training showed that when a person has this certainty and unreserved self-esteem, he has the total love and support of those around him.

We now have nine certified rebirthers in the world. The list will increase as time goes on. The first nine are:

1. Leonard Orr
2. Diane Hinterman
3. Bobby Birdsall
4. Fred Lehrman
5. Steven Kamp
6. Sondra Ray
7. Bill Chappelle
8. Bob Mandell
9. Jim Morningstar

The Rebirthee

Regardless of how talented the rebirther is, it is really *you* who has to do the rebirthing. You can rebirth yourself alone. It is, however, wise, pleasurable and appropriate to form a relationship with a rebirther. A qualified rebirther increases the efficiency and safety of the rebirth experience. Later, after you have had a breathing release, you will be able to rebirth yourself safely without the rebirther present. Leonard worked on his own rebirth for over five years and didn't complete it until he trained a dozen rebirthers and had them rebirth him. His conclusion: Certain aspects, because of the complexity of the mind and the time between birth and rebirth, are frightening to face without the presence of someone who is experienced and capable. Rebirthing is a regression to infancy, and a characteristic of the infant is a need to be cared for. It is not practical to rebirth yourself until you have passed through the infancy stage. Leonard has seen many people dissolve the birth trauma in five sessions or less, while it took him years to do it alone.

If you are normal and well-adjusted, and if you are willing to take maximum responsibility for your participation in the rebirth, then you will probably be able to wipe out the substance of your birth trauma and its effects in one to five sessions and will establish a new relationship to your divine spiritual energy. If you devote your complete attention and will to the rebirthing, it is easy. If you are essentially unwilling to face the truth about yourself, it may take a hundred sessions to do the same thing. Paradoxically, fear of failure prevents success. A willingness to face things is characteristic of successful people.

Ideally, you will be able to attend a rebirth seminar, which will help you to establish rapport with the rebirther and to gain enough information to prevent surprises that may entrap the mind and slow down the process. The rebirthing seminar enables you to get much more value from your rebirth experience and to reduce the number of rebirths necessary to reach completion. You will be instructed to read Dr. LeBoyer's book, *Birth Without Violence,* which will stimulate the memory of your own birth. You will be given certain affirmations to write that will help to create safety in your mind (like "I can now breathe fully and freely"). You will also learn how physical immortality relates to rebirthing and to your life.

After selecting your rebirther, you will be expected to agree to continue sessions until you achieve the breathing release and are past the infancy stage. Your relationship with your first rebirther is very important, so be sure that there is good rapport between you and the person you select. Later you may choose to have another rebirther because of some special affinity.

Rebirthing can be done in groups, but it is much preferable to do it individually so that you can have all the loving attention that you deserve and did not get in your original birth. Leonard has experimented with doing fifty to a hundred people at once by having them work in pairs. He feels that this is not ideal. However, the results are too beneficial to ignore. Because of my work in loving relationships training, I especially enjoy rebirthing couples. Watching each other go through this process produced a whole new level of understanding and depth of love.

Leonard is eager to give everyone an opportunity to heal their breathing mechanism, to learn to breath fully and freely, and to experience the cleansing and healing power of divine energy in the physical body. However, at this point, we feel that rebirthing in groups compromises the quality of the experience. Leonard is totally dedicated to maintaining the quality of the experience and therefore has dedicated himself to training high quality rebirthers that probably in the end will expand the work more quickly than mass rebirthings. If Leonard dedicated himself to groups of fifty to one hundred people he could do perhaps ten or twenty thousand people a year, however. We currently plan to train approximately five hundred rebirthers a year; those well-trained rebirthers can rebirth over twenty thousand people a month; so even mathematically, staying totally focused on the quality and purity of the training of rebirthers is the most effective way to influence the results. In other words, raising the quality of your own consciousness is still and will forever be the most efficient way to save the world.

When we started writing this book, we thought: Wouldn't it be wonderful if we could write a book that would enable a person to rebirth himself? Now that it is written we have rebirthed over ten thousand persons and have formed the following conclusions:

1. This chapter, and the whole book, will rebirth you on some level. This chapter may induce a rebirthing cycle. This chapter may eliminate a rebirthing cycle that you had spontaneously once, without understanding what it was.

2. Because of the instrumentality, safety, and spiritual reciprocity that takes place during a rebirthing, it is impossible for this book to substitute for what we call a complete rebirthing cycle in the presence of a trained professional rebirther. Doing it alone deprives you of the love and support you might receive from the rebirthers. No book can give you this.

Our purpose then is to see that you get the most from your rebirthing process. There are two things to consider:

1. One is your understanding of the process. Re-reading this chapter during the rebirthing cycle is invaluable. It will increase the efficiency with which you master the rebirthing process in your own mind and body. It could save you months of discomfort and mental anguish.

2. Since we have trained over five hundred rebirthers now, they will be rebirthing approximately ten thousand people a month. This success may attract others who will present themselves as rebirthers. Hopefully we will give you sufficient information so that you may protect yourself should you find yourself in the company of a charlatan.

We are discussing these points at the beginning to make you aware of the power of rebirthing so that if a spontaneous rebirth occurs, you will not be overly concerned and not overreact. The correct thing to do is to breathe in a relaxed rhythm if illness, fear, or discomfort occur. Even if it is familiar and you think you know what it is, breathe and relax through it, and if it persists call a rebirther.

As rebirthing and other forms of spiritual enlightenment become more widespread throughout society, more and more people will be spontaneously induced into a rebirth experience by the psychic safety produced by enlightened people around them. The ideas in this chapter will create feelings of safety in your mind and body and, although nothing may happen while you are reading it, after mentally digesting these ideas, you may have a spontaneous rebirth while making love, resting in bed, listening to beautiful music or watching TV. It is important not to panic and do harm to yourself. The rebirth phenomenon is totally safe if you just relax and breath in a relaxed manner. A common denominator in birth trauma is fear of irreparable damage. Most people resent leaving the womb and therefore experience irreparable damage in being denied readmission. Since they don't integrate the experience of birth into their consciousness and understand it, they go through life with a constant fear of irreparable damage. Unfortunately the subconscious can take this fear and turn it into a causative expectation. When you study the impact in human emotions of the birth trauma, you can see what it causes everywhere in human behavior. For example, we noted a statistical correlation in people who are slapped on the fanny at birth and people who later have rear ended automobile accidents. Many forms of crime, victim consciousness, failure and illness can be traced to this fear of irreparable damage.

Whenever you experience intense anxiety, fear of harm, or irreparable damage, find a safe place and sit or lie down, relax and breathe. If you are working with a well-trained rebirther, you will quickly understand the dynamics of all this and learn how to handle it with ease. Until then, we offer these guidelines.

Finally, it is impossible for a book to substitute for the dialogue of a rebirth seminar or a harmonious successful relationship with a rebirther. On the other hand, this book will explain things that you will never have time to get in seminars or in that relationship. It will make a relationship to a rebirther a million times more efficient. For most of you, the book will shed valuable light on disturbances that trouble and terrify you. It is our hope that you will take time to meditate on these ideas and utilize them in your spiritual evolution. Reading this chapter aloud to a friend is a very powerful experience.

The Ideal Rebirthing Sequence

Leonard has many of his personal rebirth clients go through what we might call the ideal rebirthing sequence. The first, dry session is a powerful cycle which usually contains paralysis that people go through rather efficiently because they are willing to follow instructions. The second session is four to ten days later, after a person has had time to rest and integrate the first one. It is the heaviest and longest because the rebirthee is willing to let go completely and feel safe enough to permit the energy to overwhelm him and do its healing work.

The third one is what Leonard calls the scary one, because the rebirth seems to be going smoothly and all at once the throat constricts or internal fluids are generated that cause the rebirthee to choke and strangle. There is fear of death from clogged air passages and inability to breathe. When the rebirther reminds the rebirthee that it is a *memory* and encourages him to relax, then the panic subsides and is breathed out in several cycles. The third session is more intense, but usually shorter, than number two.

The fourth session is what you might call a re-run of parts of all three, but also has unique characteristics of its own. Throughout the fifth one, which can also be described as a re-run, the rebirthee is able to breathe smoothly and rhythmically without fear. It usually takes half as long as number two, for example. This is the time to start wet rebirthings, which are pleasurable and interesting.

Rebirthing Fees

Rebirthing is a divine gift—and so is everything else we have in this world. It is reasonable that those who become professional rebirthers be supported by their work. Thirty-five to fifty dollars is a reasonable fee for one rebirth session at the time of this writing, although inflation may necessitate increases in the future. It is very important for the financial agreement between the rebirther and rebirthee to be worked out in advance, so that a person is free to complete the process. Many people think our suggested fee is too *in*expensive, considering that rebirthing is the most effective, fastest technique of self-improvement that we know.

If you think you need to get rebirthed free, state that in advance and find a rebirther who is willing to do it. The policy of Leonard and his associates (Rebirth International) is to do a certain percentage of their work without pay. Every rebirther has a certain scholarship quota. Bartering of energy and talents is also sometimes possible. The important factor is that the agreement reflect mutual respect and genuine commitment to and support of one another. Rebirthers are willing to give it away and we are willing to be prospered abundantly from our work. Either way, our primary motive is service. The substance of our work is raising the quality of human consciousness.

Follow Up to Rebirthing

If you decide to open Pandora's box and get rebirthed, then you should know that there is an easy way and a hard way. The easy way is to take the advice we give you here and be part of a spiritual community. The hard way is to stay alone, without all the advantages and techniques a spiritual community has to offer. The easy way is to participate in all the related seminars possible and take them over and over until you feel totally safe. It took me at least a year to absorb all the concepts Leonard had to offer, at least a year to integrate all the reactions from my rebirthings, and at least a year to experience the real benefits of physical immortality. I now know the feeling of being "on the right side of the law," where everything happens effortlessly and I can easily and quickly manifest my thoughts in the physical universe. I'll outline how I did it. You are welcome to follow my path. It was the most efficient one I saw at the time. Now we have much improved and speeded up the path for your convenience as you can see by our forty-day plan, etc.

1. Spiritual Psychology Seminar

This was the first seminar I ever took. It is excellent. We used to use it as preparation for rebirthing before we invented the rebirthing seminar. Now you have the fortune to read some data from this seminar right in this book. However, being in the seminar itself is so beneficial, that you will want to take it again and again.

2. Self-Analysis Seminar

This needs to be experienced and is not included in the data of this book because the seminar leader works with his psychic intuitive power to assist you to discover just what is your *personal law*. Then he will assist you to use affirmations to change this important law to something positive that will work for you in your life and to erase negative patterns. It is very powerful.

3. Physical Immortality Seminar

I took this seminar eight times in a row even though I had worked out a great deal of my unconscious death urge prior to meeting Leonard. (I did it alone which was definitely the "low road" and the hard way.) In this seminar I always released tremendous sensations in my body. I was just fascinated to see how my body would react differently each time . . . and to note at which points I "went unconscious" and didn't hear what was being said. Every time I attended I felt better and happier and healthier.

4. Money Seminar

I slept through the whole seminar or "went unconscious," so I took this over and over. It was hard for me to absorb because I had something wired up about money and death. I felt this seminar really assisted me financially. Without it, I might have had trouble making money because I was so into infancy. It is important to understand how the other concepts of birth trauma and the unconscious death urge affect your money case.

5. Affirmations Seminar

We don't teach this seminar much anymore because the technique is covered in depth in my book, *I Deserve Love*. But I want to stress here how very important it is that you do absorb the affirmations technique once you start rebirthing. The affirmations technique is the source of mental health (along with correct breathing, of course) and mastering your personal reality. Affirmations got me through whatever came up for me between rebirths. I was so thankful for this life-saver that I wrote a whole book on the subject. If you understand and use affirmations you can dissolve anything or create anything.

6. Spiritual Healing Seminar

This is the way to understand that you are in control of your body and can cure anything. In it you learn how to clear up any physical problems, especially when you find it inconvenient to get rebirthed. It is important to have these techniques to go along with rebirthing.

7. Spiritual Literature Seminar

I read as many spiritual books as I could get my hands on the first year. This is very helpful to keep the process going. There are some that Leonard recommends that are more beneficial than others. What we have done is try to read a book every week and then get together to discuss what we read. (See the list of recommended readings at the end of this book.)

8. Consultations

One of the benefits of a spiritual community is that you can always find a therapist or consultant with whom you can get your head clear between rebirths. If you do not have a professional, you can co-counsel with a friend by doing half-hour trades of listening to each other for free. At Theta House in San Francisco, the consultation fee is $50, and I feel it is well worth it. I got tremendous value out of seeing Leonard or Kyle (who have been my consultants whenever my boyfriends got tired of handling my case) whenever things got very heavy. I make myself available as a consultant for my rebirthees whenever possible, because many times they just need to discuss what has come up for them since their rebirth and they do not feel emotionally ready to have another rebirth at that time. The same goes for the graduates of my Loving Relationships Training. The training is very powerful and often graduates need one or two private sessions to get assistance in handling the emotional material that was stimulated.

9. The One-Year Seminar

Of all, this is the single most beneficial and safest place to "process." Here you will find a group of thirty-fifty people who meet together once or twice a month for a year. All the ideas from other seminars are incorporated and you are helped to put them into practice in your own life. The wonderful thing about the One-Year Seminar is that you can work out your infancy and family case with all the members, since they are the same every month. You can "set up" people as your mother, father, sister or brother and resolve those relationships safely. In Leonard's very first One-Year Seminar we went through phenomenal growth by having the freedom to do that with each other. I once went into a complete primal on the floor after Leonard instructed me to crawl around the room like a toddler. My friends comforted me afterwards with love and warm milk which they fed me with a spoon. I liked having the freedom to "say anything" and feel safe. After all, especially in those days, you couldn't tell just anyone, "My birth trauma is getting heavy and my death urge is up and I feel like vomiting every morning." It is also in the One-Year Seminar where you learn to become your own guru, along with getting practice leading seminars and learning how to do spiritual healing.

10. *The Loving Relationships Training*

In some areas, there are evening seminars on relationships. However, the most comprehensive one is the weekend training I developed, which covers all the Theta principles we teach and applies them directly to relationships. Actually, all there *is* is relationships, and when I finally got that concept and also saw how people suffer in relationships, I decided to devote a great portion of my life to this matter. I have been inspired by the phenomenal results in my graduates' lives. It warms my heart tremendously when graduates tell me they were easily able to find a mate with whom they are happy, by using the techniques I teach in the training. And that their relationships are continuing to work . . . and that their love is increasing daily . . . and that their lives are unfolding. They thank me profusely. I silently thank Leonard and the Spirit for getting me to the place where I can share this knowledge.

So now you see the path I took, in the order I did it. It is not necessary to follow this order. You can start at ten and work the other way. I have tried to put a little of each in my training. So you could do that for an overview, and then study each area in depth afterwards. You can do it any way you like. The point is that these seminars work and they do assist you in handling your "case," as we call it lovingly. I feel it would be unethical not to mention these things that are available for you, as we are sincerely interested in making it all as pleasurable as possible for you. So as an "old timer" in the rebirthing business I am glad to say that we have now made it easier for you and we will continue to improve and expedite the whole process of unlocking the birth-death cycle so that you can get into bliss as fast as possible.

Rick's Story

It is probably worth recording that I first got rebirthed, as it is called, because I wanted to make money. Teaching people how to prosper themselves and others is one of the things Leonard Orr does in his Theta seminar program. It happened that during this particular seminar a rebirth was scheduled for the entire group. Only three of us had never gone through the process, and we all decided to try it. I was interested and well-disposed towards it because a friend of mine, Peggy Utne, had visited me the night before, just after having what she described as a "terrific" rebirth with Leonard. Her whole breathing had been changed, she said, and possibly her whole being with it. She was glowing even more than usual, and a certain very subtle awkwardness which she usually wore had been lifted entirely. Come to think of it, she had been the one who'd told me about the money seminar.

Leonard asked for qualified rebirthers to assist the three of us so that we could go in separate rooms and have our first rebirthing privately. Dave, from Milwaukee, said that he would do mine. My first choice had naturally been the most interesting-looking female there; Dave looked OK, though I didn't quite believe his satisfied smile.

The First Rebirth

I lie down in a small New York bedroom and take off my shirt. This is so he can watch my breathing, Dave tells me, as if to reassure me. He asks me if I have any considerations or questions, which I don't. After all, as a New Age journalist, sixties veteran, and practicing Buddhist, I've been through more than a few trips and I figure I can handle this one.

As I start breathing through my mouth, which is open wider than usual, according to rebirthing practice, I feel a tingling, not unpleasant, above my knees. Suddenly it's hard to breath. My chest feels like an iron band around my lungs. Dave pushes my jaw down, gently. It feels tight, and I tell him so, but the words come out so strangled that I have to repeat them more than once. I can see that, he says. My feet tingle, tiny pins and needles, and then turn solid as wood. It's uncanny how fast it is all happening, and just from this simple way of breathing: *pulling* the inhale and then just releasing the exhale. My hands, too, turn to wood. I am sweating now, thinking, this stuff is powerful—and therefore dangerous. I try crossing my hands over my chest, looking for a position that will ease the pain. There is none. Keep breathing, says David. There seems to be no space between the cells of my body. The feeling is not just numb and wooden now, but there is contraction, a paralysis pressing in, an implosion. Desperately, I try to relax and escape the pain. I can't.

I can't stand it, I try to say. My open jaws are clenched so tight Dave can't understand the words. The muscles of my hands are frozen into claws, and there is something prehistoric, fossil-like, about my posture. I move my hands, throbbing with pain, over my head, this way, that way, but it doesn't help. The truth is I *can't* relax. Beneath my sweating skin, stretched taut as a drum, the muscles are contracting by themselves.

I know it feels like you have to relax, says Dave, but the only way to do it is to stay with the breathing. As far as I'm concerned he's out of his mind, but I try to follow his advice, since he got me into this. What had started out as another interesting experiment, another more or less valuable experience to add to my storehouse of spiritual-psychological tales, has turned into more pain than I bargained for. It hurts like hell.

"Do you usually try to push, to plow through things?" asks Dave.

"No," I say in a voice that hardly seems my own. "I usually try to ignore them."

"Well," David answers, "you can't ignore *this*."

I have no argument with this. There is obviously no way to avoid your own birth, or, by extension, anything else that's yours by birthright. I stay with the breathing and with the pain.

Every now and then Dave touches me lightly, above the knee, on my ankle, my chest, and reminds me not to push the air out. Somehow, without my noticing it, the blocks of my hands and feet start tingling, bubbles of feeling arise, and then fade, dissolve, and disappear. Without planning it I sneak a deep relaxed out-breath, a simple and profound sigh, which opens the door of my chest. "Ah, that was a good one," says Dave. He sounds pleased, as if it were his breath too.

My eyes are half open. The soft afternoon light washes pleasurably in. Waves of intense pleasure roll through my body, waves of light, of feeling, of movement. I have as little to do with them as the ocean with its waves: they just rise and fall, rise and fall. Ah, pleasure—the other side of pain, I think. Dave feels it too. It illuminates the narrow little bedroom. The light is rosy through the drawn shade. The oceanic streamings flow, reach a peak, ebb, and slowly subside.

There is still a little tingling, and a few hard knots in my body. I want it to be over, now that it's already happened. "Take your time," says Dave. It's true, I see, that I am always in a hurry, speedy. I rest. More pleasure-waves, and a light bubbly euphoria. Dave leaves, and I notice a sweet odor in the room, a little too sweet and heavy, familiar and yet unplaceable. I get up, piss, then walk out into the larger room where people are scattered around, sprawled casually on the rug as if they were lying on a beach, after the group rebirth. I see Leonard talking to someone, and a flash, a spark of acknowledgment, jumps from his eyes to mine. I thank him and go out to the terrace, where I swing in a hammock, easily and peacefully, back and forth, and there is nowhere else to go.

Later, after an hour or two of feeling light and good, I come down, as we say. I feel hot and irritable and tired, which is not surprising since I'd had about three hours sleep the night before. I argue with Sara, who had had *her* first rebirth screaming and crying in the room next to mine, about whether to go dancing downtown. She wants to go to the Ocean Club. I decide to let her go on alone while I stay home to quietly absorb the rebirthing experience. Dancing, she says, is her way of absorbing a new experience. Yet we both want to be together—it is that kind of argument.

When I go out on Christopher Street, a summer night crowd stands around a man playing a very, very mellow sax for all he is worth. I wonder what I am so uptight about. And what are all these people doing out late Sunday night? Then I remember it is Saturday night, not Sunday, and the next morning is not a Monday morning. For some reason this gives me a great sense of relief. I go back down to the subway to go dancing.

Second Rebirth

The next day I had lunch with Leonard during the seminar break. I told him the following experience, which, even though it had occurred fifteen years ago, continued still fresh, or at least present, in my mind.

For a number of months, fifteen years ago, I would become paralyzed and unable to breathe when in the twilight state between waking and sleeping, usually when very tired. I would slip into this state and be unable to move or breathe. The harder I tried to breathe, and to move, the more panicked I became, and the stronger the paralysis became. It got so that I was afraid to go to sleep when I felt psychically exhausted, since this was the time I seemed most susceptible.

One evening I was talking about this problem with my girlfriend. She suggested that the next time I felt the dream approaching I should not try to wake and move, but I should just relax and watch it. She also pointed out that if my breathing stopped for a dangerously long time my body would automatically wake up.

I began to drift into the familiar twilight state almost as soon as we stopped talking, only this time I did not resist it. A loud voice, curiously amplified—a man's voice—spoke to me from the far corner of the room. The voice told me, in some detail, what the causes of my paralysis were. At that point I turned and told Anne, who was reading on the bed next to me, what the voice had told me. Something about what I said upset or saddened her, and she began to cry. Then she got up and went into the bathroom. At that moment I woke up.

Anne was lying on the bed next to me, reading. I asked her if I had just told her something, and if she had been crying. She said that I hadn't told her anything. I had been sleeping, and had just now awakened. I tried to remember the words of the voice, but they were fading fast, as dreams will. I seemed to remember something about women, and being wrapped and held tightly as a child; but I wasn't sure, since one of my own theories about the causes of the paralysis had to do with being too tightly confined as an infant. But I did have a strong feeling of respect, even admiration, for the resourcefulness and intelligence of my mind in keeping its secrets from itself.

There was one more interesting thing about this experience, I told Leonard over coffee. Even though I could never remember the exact words from the dream, I never again was paralyzed in my sleep.

Leonard thought this was an interesting example of a spontaneous rebirth experience. It was, now that I thought about it, similar to what I had gone through the day before, at least in spirit. Leonard asked me if my mother had taken much anesthetic when I was born; I wasn't sure, but I said I would ask her. And then I thought I placed the odor of whatever it was that had been lingering in my nostrils like an over-ripe bouquet of flowers since the rebirth: chloroform.

The second rebirth took place that afternoon, along with everybody else, on the carpeted floor of a Holiday Inn conference room. Apparently I no longer needed special attention. The second rebirth proceeded much like the first one. I thought at first that nothing would happen, but as I kept on breathing through my mouth the same sensations, and lack of sensations, and pain, occurred in the same parts of my body. At one point I felt a blockage of energy, like static, around my wrist, and looked down to see that I had forgotten to remove my metal Tibetan bracelet. As soon as Dave helped me take it off the blockage opened. The streamings in my body were pleasurable, more pleasant than euphoric this time, and I was able to play with my own breathing, pacing myself. I could feel my heart beat freely in my chest. I continued working with the breathing and as I tried to breath more deeply I felt my chest refuse to open. Then I began choking until I brought up and spit out a small glob of phlegm. I looked at Dave and felt at one with him; he seemed included in the lightness which, rather than my skin, seemed to be the boundary of my body. I reflected that this experience, whether or not it was connected to my actual historical birth, was valuable in itself, and thought, for some reason, that it would be useful training in how to die. Birth and death, I thought, is a revolving door.

A few days later I telephoned my mother and asked her if she had had much anesthetic when I was born. "And how!" she said. They had really dosed her, so much so that she had resolved to have her next child, my sister, by the then-revolutionary method of natural childbirth.

The Next Two Rebirths

Third Rebirth, dry, Theta House, San Francisco
Same slight smell—as of sulpher, or ether, or anesthetic,
as before, in my previous rebirths.
Less paralysis, hands of foam rubber.
I had prepared, it seemed, by stopping smoking
days before, taking deep breaths instead of cigarettes.

I felt resistance, nausea in the solar plexus.
Love it, love yourself, said Paul,
Anything connected with it?
Felt a sadness.
Love it, breathe into it, said Paul.
Memories of 14? 11? Parents splitting,

mother talking urgently
on telephone, crying later.
I'm playing catch, first depression—
Out of it, into myself.
Breathe into your ankles, your feet. Your knees.
Get the answer to a problem with a piece on Holistic Health
I'm working on—
but also bothered by the thought that I can't pay attention
to the experience I'm having now.
Very light floaty feeling now.
Body feels *real* light, just slight nausea in the pit of stomach.
Breathing goes *all* the way down.
Eyes closed.
Last faint tinglings in hand.

Fourth Rebirth

The earlier appointment had been cancelled. I felt slightly
relieved, since I was more than a little nervous about going into
the tank for the first time.

It was hard to remember the details, even just a half-hour after
the rebirth. Hand and foot paralysis started rather quickly. I
reached the first stage, and realized that the feelings were much
more powerful than in the previous one. The pit of my stomach
hurt, and then the whole center of my stomach become a little
vortex of speed and anxiety. I spit up phlegm a few times. Paul
directed my breathing. The pain of the paralysis around my hands
and feet was intense, and my central thought was, "I want it to be
over." It simply hurt too much. I had thought that because of the
relative ease of the last time this time would be easier. The
paralysis abated somewhat, but then Paul asked for more rapid
breathing, and it came back even more, my body spread-eagled,
and then contracted in again.

It is hard to remember, as I said, even now, just an hour afterwards, what it felt like—there were great flashes of consecutive

darkness, like doors closing one after another. I wanted it to be over, and said as much. "You have to love it," said Paul, and I mentally asked "How?" But, of course, there is no "how" to love. I felt a sadness again, this time like a ring round my jaw, and tried to breathe into it. I couldn't hold my head straight. Like a baby's it swayed to and fro, or like a flower on a stalk in the wind. I went down again into the warm water making moans, groans that echoed like Oms in a gigantic watery cathedral; after a while Paul suggested I stop the sounds. I began to feel very good, but tired, and thanked Paul and the assistant. On coming up I had an impulse to take her breast in my mouth, but I let it pass. My lower back, fifth dorsal, felt unsupported, so I told Paul, and he supported me there, which made my stomach relax more.

I was dizzy climbing out of the tub, a little woozy. Lying down, with no cover since my body felt so warm and alive, I felt a sadness gradually rise from my chest to my jaw. Breathing moved way down into my belly. A sudden flash of thought crossed my face. Paul asked me what it had been. I caught it. It was money. We talked about it for a while, how I felt I didn't deserve it. "Who does deserve it?" said Paul. I thought about that for a while. "The people with credentials," I said.

Then I remembered a time, which I told Paul about, when I had slept through an exam while I was on probation in college. Missing the exam caused me to be suspended from college for a year; I never went back; no credentials. The incident occurred around the same time I had had my dreams of paralysis. It seemed a way, I told Paul, of proving to the world how lazy I was. I still, in fact, sleep through the beginnings of the day, wasting most mornings.

Plans for my book, and ideas for articles were bubbling up in my mind. Paul asked if I always lived in the future. It seemed to me that I did. So we talked about that, about how that might be related to my wanting it to be over and finished. The resistance of fear to pleasure is pain, I saw, and I saw also how that is related to my not living in one place, not concentrating on one thing, not finishing projects . . .

"Why not rest here, and give yourself pleasure," suggested Paul.

OK, I thought, but I've really got to be going.

I left for Boulder the next day, still not smoking, breathing from the pit of my stomach at whim.

Rick Fields

Rebirther Comments

None of Rick's rebirths show breathing release yet. Now that we have perfected the process, we usually have five or ten dry rebirths which in most cases produce a breathing release. Then after the breathing release, a person get either a holistic energy cycle, or no energy and just realizations and memories of birth, whether it is wet or dry. Using water before a breathing release usually causes a person to need twice as many rebirths. After a breathing release, primal feelings can surface to consciousness physically or psychologically at any time; however the person has the ability in his breath to literally pump out any unpleasantness that may arise.

We allowed Rick to do a wet rebirth before completing his breathing release for two reasons: one is because he desired to very strongly; the other is because the water sometimes breaks up the "anesthesia number" faster. As he described, his paralysis was heavier in the water, which indicates that he had more fear.

Wet rebirths are now like a final exam. They provide the rebirthee with an opportunity to re-run the key parts of his birth memories and sometimes stimulate other important primal material.

Gary's Story

First Rebirth

As an American middle-class growth junkie, I'm always open to hearing about new ways to "clean up my act," as they say. So, when I overheard some of my friends talking about rebirthing I tuned in instantly. The name of the process alone was enough to intrigue me. Besides, if there's one thing I've learned from all the hours and hours of processing done in various enlightenment games, it's how to say yes!

Contrary to the popular style of choosing one's rebirther on the basis of intuition, my rebirther chose me. Her name was Isara White and a more perfect mother-substitute there could not have been. Isara is soft, warm, tender, loving, open, motherly . . . and she has big, soft breasts.

Isara also was willing to let me assist, or sit in at, the rebirthing of my friend, office manager and business partner, Claudia, before I had my first rebirth. This is not standard procedure, but we both agreed that I could handle it and that in my case it would be excellent preparation for my first rebirth. I got very "plugged in" to Claudia's rebirth, as I thought I might. A lot of sadness came up for her and since I'm a sucker for women crying anyway I resonated perfectly with her anguish and grief. I left Isara's house that afternoon on the verge of tears, barely able to breathe, and experiencing trepidation at the prospect of my own rebirth and next afternoon.

The next day I lay on the soft carpet at Isara's, trying to relax, and being mildly annoyed at the incessant traffic noise outside the window above my head. Claudia was there, at my request and with Isara's approval. I read aloud from *Birth Without Violence* for about ten minutes—although this was entirely unnecessary, as I had been having numerous and intensely vivid visual and auditory flashbacks to my birth since I had attended Isara's rebirth seminar one week previously. The moment had arrived, I thought. This is it. I am ready.

Instantly, in a time-lapse yet timeless filmstrip, I reviewed all the times in my life I had taken irrevocable action. The time I jumped off the high rocks into the pool at Waimea falls, Hawaii, my first acid trip, the times I got married. Here I was again, on the precipice of a new and exciting experience, knowing intuitively that as a result of it, I would be changed forever. In a very childlike way I said to myself something I hadn't said in years: "One, two, three, here goes nothin'." Isara, lying beside me, interrupted me after two breaths and said "There's just one thing I want you to know before we begin; I'm really feeling a lot of love for you right now, right here in my heart." Her hand was over her breast to illustrate this and as she looked at me I experienced her love in every bone, fiber and tissue of my body. I was touched deeply and thoroughly by her love, and in that moment I knew total safety and certainty. I knew that I could withstand or sustain absolutely anything. Her love was all over me like a blanket. And I surrendered.

In less than five deep rhythmic breaths I was beginning to tingle and hum in my hands and face. A pungent, yet not unpleasant, metallic taste appeared in my mouth, nose and throat. I had the image of being carried along gently yet powerfully on a river. My now more rapid breaths were the waves and troughs over which I rollercoastered, inexorably carried downstream toward a destination I could not see.

I checked in. Isara lying beside me, her hand placed tenderly on my heaving chest. Yes. OK. Claudia sitting nearby watching me intently, not breathing, "plugged in." Yes. Room still here, traffic noise outside. Right. Furniture all in the same place. Pictures still hung in the same locations. Yes, everything is OK. But wait!! I just saw all this with my eyes closed! Something is weird here. But I don't have time to ruminate on all this. The river beckons.

Back on the waves and troughs I have the sudden realization that I am no longer in control. I look around. It's true. No oars, no paddles, no outboard. I'm breathing in a rich deep rhythmic racehorse pant and I'm totally out of control. I couldn't stop this if I wanted to. A moment of panic flashes by. I recall a movie I saw years and years ago which starred Marilyn Monroe. In it her husband, distraught and jealous, kills himself by plunging over Niagara Falls, clinging to a frail piece of wood. That's it! I've been wondering why the waves and troughs have been getting deeper and steeper. I'm approaching the rapids. I'm nearing the falls and there isn't a goddamned thing I can do. Suddenly I know I'm going to die and I'm mighty pissed about it all. My breathing has reached high gear. My back arches up in a paroxysm of pain and anger. My throat clamps down and instinctively I gape my mouth wide open. I'm a fish thrown high and dry. Gasping. Taking that last breath before the plunge into the roaring chaos below. I look around one more time. Isara and Claudia are whooping and jumping for joy. Isara is saying something like: "Oh wow, this is the breathing release, Claudia! Keep breathing!!" Breathing release, shit!! I'm dying, you motherfuckers, and you're excited! Confusion, bewilderment. Followed by oblivion. I arch up in one final glorious spasm. No pictures. No emotions. No thoughts. My last conscious memory is the dying climactic strains of Wagner's Love-Death theme from *Tristan und Isolde.* Then it's over.

Over. Yes, and I'm over too. Over the gap. Over the chasm. Over the abyss. Over the bridge. But there *was* no bridge! I did it like Evel Knievel! Catapulted over the whole gaping hole. But I made the entire distance. And without a parachute! I'm smiling. In one moment out of time I am transformed from a chugging locomotive. Thirty-two years of hauling heavily laden freight cars up a never-ending incline. Now I am free. Free and free forever. I am free.

Isara moves in close and snuggles up to me. She listens to my breathing. Each breath fills my entire torso from the base of my balls to the tip of my curly head. Those elusive full free pinnacle-peak breaths I only used to be able to grab every so often are now ordinary, common. My mind is reeling. I don't remember anything. What happened to the pictures of my birth, I wonder. I'm so used to seeing a movie. Screw it. I notice, almost casually, that I'm in bliss. Claudia comes over and lies down next to me also. I am surrounded by love and warm yielding femininity. Theirs . . . and my own. With both women tucked under my arms and pressed closely I begin to softly weep. Isara and Claudia are gushing with pride for my triumph. I am gushing tears of elation, feeling the intensity and purity of their love for me.

Sometime later, as I climb slowly and carefully to my feet, Isara is repeating to herself for the third time that I represent her graduation in rebirthing from a trainee to a professional. I am, she says, her very first first-appointment breath release. She is ecstatic. Claudia is ecstatic. I am ecstatic. We are all deliriously ga-ga. Isara is now a first-rate postgraduate rebirther. And as for me . . . well, I've been on what Leonard calls "the right side of the law" ever since.

Second Rebirth

Not too many days after my first rebirth in Honolulu, I found myself in San Francisco taking in some R&R. My partner, Claudia, thought it best that I leave our business for a short while and integrate my first rebirthing experience. I disagreed. She insisted. I resisted. She persisted, saying that the company would not fall apart without me and that she would look after everything.

I found her intention to be higher than mine the next morning when I arrived at work early and found the door locked and the key removed from its usual hiding place. Since rebirthing had taught me to surrender, I shrugged my shoulders and flew out that night.

As a part of my R&R I had made it a goal to visit Theta House in San Francisco and look around. The effects of that first rebirthing had had such a dramatic and (you'll pardon the expression) inspiring effect on my psyche that I was, even at this early date, looking at the possibility of becoming a rebirther myself. Besides, Isara had told me that she thought I thought I would make a great one.

I made inquiries in the Theta Office and was told that Bobby Birdsall, one of the five Certified Rebirthers, was currently doing a weekend intensive rebirthing right there in Theta House and that he would be back from lunch shortly and would be happy to talk with me about being a rebirther. I was in luck. Oops! I mean I was on the right side of the law again.

A short time later, in swaggered a short, cocky little stick of dynamite who identified himself as Bobby. At first glance I couldn't put my finger on who he reminded me of. Then it came to me: He was a well-proportioned mixture of Mick Jagger, Napoleon, Dustin Hoffman and Mahatma Ghandi. I didn't tell him that.

We talked briefly about the life of a rebirther and the more we talked the more my image of a rebirther was blown away. I had it figured out that all rebirthers were kind, loving, warm, tender, soft and had big breasts. Bobby Birdsall didn't fit my rebirther role model at all during that first encounter, and that was only the beginning.

In the course of the discussion I was invited by Bobby and his assistant, Pam Whitney, to stick around for the weekend rebirth intensive. Pam, being bright, buoyant and big-breasted, came a lot closer to my carefully constructed model of a rebirther so I agreed to do the weekend with them. "To be a good rebirther," they said, "first you have to learn to be a good rebirthee."

When I arrived at Theta House next morning we were all ushered upstairs to the large attic which has been comfortably remodeled into a meeting room. From the ceiling is suspended a most unusual patchwork quilt of huge proportions and rich colors. It is bordered all around by a thick hem which gives it the appearance of being very organic. I was fascinated by this terrible thing. I couldn't take my eyes off it. I had seen things like it in anatomy texts. Horrible gooey things. Membranes. Peritoneums. (Gasp.) Placentas! That was it! It looked exactly like a huge dangling afterbirth. I got dizzy and had to sit down. Jesus. We hadn't even started the seminar yet and already I was sinking into the doo-doo of my birth trauma again. Vivid visuals of my birth began to flash by.

Being covert, I didn't let on to anyone that all this was happening. I was in relatively good shape however, because, having had my breathing release, I could center myself quickly with a few unobtrusive deep sighs. Pam and Bobby soon came unwittingly to my rescue and started the seminar by having each one of us introduce ourselves. I found, much to my delight, that I was in the company of seven other rebirthees, all female! I lightened up at the prospect of having several little girl nurserymates to play with that day. Turning my back on the wretched glop of tissue hanging from the ceiling, I gave my full attention to Bobby.

I have never in my life known anyone to impart so much valuable information about rebirthing, birth trauma, the five biggies, spiritual enlightenment and physical immortality while talking about street fighting in New York, riding motorcycles, going to jail, living out of garbage cans and being an orphan: all of which Bobby has done. Right after lunch we were all back upstairs, selecting our spots on the floor like third-graders ready for nap time. With everyone snugly wrapped in blankets and starting to breathe deeply, I began again to read aloud from *Birth Without Violence,* this time to the group. It didn't take too very long before I began to hear the first muffled sobs and squeaks. I was reading strongly and powerfully and clearly recreating mental images of the words in the book. Everyone was getting it totally, including me. I felt my body go nutty immediately and after six short chapters I more or less fell over backwards, pulled the blanket up tightly around my neck and sunk into it.

Meanwhile, Pam and Bobby circulated among the squirming and wheezing lumps on the floor occasionally issuing a kind word of encouragement. "Let go on the exhale"; "relax and breathe"; "take it easy on yourself"; "let go and relax"; "stay with your breathing." Things like that. From time to time Pam would come around and gently touch my forehead which by now had become so tense that it felt like the tread on a new truck tire.

Group rebirthing is very powerful stuff. A sort of domino effect occurs. One person will go into experiencing his birth and the sounds and psychic energy in the room are strong sensory and extrasensory stimuli on anyone present who has not cleaned up most or all of his birth trauma. I saw again clearly why spectators were virtually never permitted at a rebirthing session.

I was well into it by this time. I was breathing deeply and fully with my newly released breathing mechanism. I felt huge energy rushes coursing through my body. My face was contorted in a spasm of fear and anger and I felt my jaw muscles tighten and relax in turns. My breathing had become tightly-packed and laborious. The tingling in my hands increased in intensity and turned, to my utter amazement, to paralysis. I was astounded. How could this happen to me? I thought I had had my breathing release. What kind of shit was this? One hand reached over under the blanket and blindly groped for the other. It jerked away in shock. My hand had the unmistakable feel of supersoft baby skin! Even the tiny wrinkles were there. I had heard that many physiological phenomena were re-experienced during rebirthing but this I had not expected.

Pictures and thoughts raced through my mind. Some obscure and meaningless, some bright and lucid. Pictures of the nursery. I heard the other rebirthees, now fully into their experiences, gasping, choking, sobbing, panting, just breathing. Something was odd. I don't remember having company in the nursery. I remember being alone in there. Alone. The word rebounded through the cavern of my mind like a note echoing through the depths of the Taj Mahal. ALONE.

The energy which had been randomly raging through my cells like a brush fire now converged in my chest, in my heart, rushed up my windpipe like hot oil and spewed forth in a burst of sound. I began wailing uncontrollably, inconsolately. Alone. I was alone. Utterly, forever, abysmally alone. Huge sobs fled from my throat. Giant tears rolled down my temples. My body squirmed and writhed. There was only anguish and pain. My hands were locked up like the claws of a boiled crab and my whole life, my whole universe was about pain and grief and anger.

"BULLSHIT!," yelled Bobby Birdsall from the other side of the room. "Quit feeling sorry for yourself, you big baby!" I was shocked out of my indulgence. He couldn't be talking to me! Not like that! Bobby appeared over me in four quick strides and stood, looking down, a sarcastic smile on his face, hands thrust down inside his pockets: "What's all dis shit about?", he asked. "Whadda you beatin' yourself up for like dat?" His New York street accent was like sandpaper on my psyche. I tried to respond to this cruel sawed-off little monster who stood towering above me but all that came out of my mouth were rude sucking sounds. I felt helpless. I felt insulted. I felt mishandled. Where was Isara?? The destruction of my "rebirther image" was complete.

Bobby then leaned over and, having gotten my attention, softened his voice and manner until he was tolerable. Bobby the marshmallow appeared. Mahatma Ghandi sans robes. Compassion flowed out of him like syrup from a maple tree. He said,

"Hey, you don't have to be so hard on yourself. Just relax. Quit beatin' yourself up. That's all over now. You never have to beat yourself up again." His words soothed me like a balm and I was so deeply touched by this tough little punk that I wept again, only this time quietly, to myself, for a short while; then I breathed the rest of the pain out and away forever.

He reached down and gently touched my forehead with his whole hand. I relaxed and realized that through all this drama and theater of the last hour there had been a thread of reality running which had never stopped or hesitated even for a moment and it was my breath. My breathing. My breath had carried me through all of it like a good sturdy boat through a storm. I loved my breath. What an odd thought.

Realizations flooded in. Free of the emotional charge attached to my birth, I was now able to clearly review it in a dispassionate and objective way. It was just a good movie now. I remembered being separated from my mother's body and being taken away to the nursery, screaming and howling. I had emerged strong, healthy, breathing and huge. I heard the doctor's voice as he watched me being carted away to the nursery. He said, "He's in fine shape now, he can take care of himself." Those were his exact words. At the moment I most needed to be in the warm, safe presence of my mother I was snatched away and placed all alone in the nursery. Those words "he can take care of himself" had become my reality. My song. My motto. My conclusion. I remembered making the decision, although on a feeling level: "OK. This is it. It looks like I'm going to have to do it all by myself."

Suddenly, like a barbershop mirror or an infinite accordion, the whole story of my life unfolded and I saw, in a moment out of time, how this decision had had an overwhelming and primary influence of my behavior. I reviewed innumerable incidents in which I opted to "do it myself." The revelation of this truth dredged up a bitter sadness over the loneliness I had endured as a result of this self-imposed fierce self-sufficiency and independence. I saw clearly the struggle my life had been because I had decided at birth never to share my burdens, tasks, endeavors or projects with others. More tears.

Then I quietly resolved to let go of this decision and free myself of it. I continued to breathe and watch with extreme elation as the whole episode slid quietly down the drain. Gradually, as time and breathing plodded on, what slight residual paralysis was left in my extremities melted away and was replaced by a pervasive glowing feeling of well-being and calmness. My environment and body became light and vibrant like a slackened guitar string gently strummed again and again.

I floated in this state until I was slightly distracted by Pam's gentle presence and soft hand stroking my head and face. What was formerly a common and familiar experience now took on a whole new dimension as I noticed that I could easily accept, even welcome, her love and attention. I would never ever again have to be alone busily "taking care of myself."

Later that afternoon as each one of us crawled dazedly out of our blanket cocoons, butterflies for sure, there was much hugging, laughing and talking. Since nearly everyone was ravenously hungry it was decided that we should all go down to Bud's for some famous ice cream. Pam drove us all, hand packed, through the streets of San Francisco, barely able to control the car. The laughter was uproarious and epidemic.

Sitting in the car gorging our hot fudge sundaes, Pam and I took turns spoon feeding each other, and as we did I reflected privately on the special significance of this simple act. Somehow it symbolized the emergence in my life of a whole new way of interacting with other human beings.

First Tub Rebirth

I arrived back in Honolulu much refreshed, relaxed and recreated. Prior to leaving for San Francisco I had set up an appointment with Isara to have my first tub rebirth three days after my arrival back in town. I was hot to go.

My first day at home I began fasting. There was something curious about this particular fast, but I couldn't quite identify the feeling. I continued fasting right up to the time of my appointment and as Claudia and I were walking up the steps toward the hot tub she remarked at how severe my fast had been. I hadn't allowed myself any juice and I had even been rationing my drinking water! A real starvation diet in every way.

Another odd set of circumstances had occurred since my return. There had been a number of upsets in my relationships during those three days, especially with women, and I had come away from work that particular day with a feeling of extreme anxiety because of some business problems regarding money and the seeming lack of it. It wasn't too long before I would be seeing the absolute perfection in these events and their direct relationship to what came up in this rebirth.

I had asked that Claudia again be present to assist. I felt very safe and at home with her and Isara there in spite of real turmoil going on inside me.

The tub we were to use was unique in that it was triangular in shape and quite small as hot tubs go. It was perfect for rebirthing because it really stimulated the feelings of closeness and confinement. This was especially the case for me since I am 6'4" and weigh 210 pounds. I bumped into the bottom and all three sides at once. It was very cozy.

The three of us undressed and sat for several minutes talking. Isara usually encourages a little open sharing before a rebirth: that is, we simply talk about whatever is on our minds at the moment. It turned out that I had a lot on my mind at that particular moment so I talked about it and got it out. It was mainly worries about work. Anyway, it went a long way to clear the air. I noticed that all during the sharing I had spent an inordinate amount of time staring at Claudia's breasts. I knew right then that something was coming up for me and it had to do with breasts. It was time to hit the water.

I put on the nose plug and snorkel. I had had a snorkel in my mouth hundreds of times before while diving in the ocean. I knew, however, that when I went under this time I was going to see things I had never seen before and they weren't going to be fishes. The water was the perfect temperature. Isara gave me a little good luck kiss and down I went. She supported my hips with her knee and hand. I float really well so it was easy. My breathing mechanism, now thoroughly conditioned, clicked into automatic rebirthing breathing mode and I was underway. Instantly my hunger pangs redoubled and dominated my consciousness. In not more than ten minutes under the water I was thoroughly regressed to the old main event and instinctively I knew it was time to come up. Isara sensed this also and eased me up and over.

My entire body was weak and shaky and I felt like a floundering whale. I came up slowly, sputtering and crying. Isara rolled me into her arms and held me, supporting my lolling head. Again my face was wrinkled into folds of anguish, my hands folded into grotesque little claws. And I was HUNGRY! Goddammit, I was hungry! Just as in San Francisco, I noticed my mouth, with a little mind of its own, making obscene sucking sounds, only this time with real desperation.

It didn't take Isara very long to figure out what was going on with me and in a flash I heard her asking me if I wanted to nurse on her breast. Even before I had time to be amazed, a wave of embarrassment rolled over me and, without thinking I shook my head emphatically, almost violently NO! I knew that she was perfectly serious and willing and my response was instantaneous. Thoughts came rushing through my mind in a torrent. All my considerations came up. Like: I can't do that. It's wrong. She is married. I only suck on women's breasts when I'm making love. Brad (Isara's husband) would hate me. Claudia is here. And on and on. I saw my whole "breast case" cracking wide open in front of my eyes. It wasn't very comfortable. Along with each of these thoughts came attendant body sensations. Everything ranging from acute embarrassment to wanton lust came up. I was confused. I was mad. I began to cry more now. Why was I denying myself that very thing I wanted so desperately, needed so totally? I was in conflict.

Isara offered me a baby bottle and a pacifier, both of which I angrily rejected. I laid there a few moments longer until the shit storm of confusion and turmoil inside my mind had subsided somewhat. Then, miraculously, from somewhere, up popped the courage to reach out into the world and ask for what I wanted.

Clumsily, I gestured toward my still sucking mouth with a crippled and pitiful-looking three fingers and the message got through. Isara confidently moved my head around and tenderly put her right breast to my mouth. I began to nurse. The contorted mask of anger and frustration which was my face, melted instantly like butter. My hands gave way and relaxed completely. I heard Claudia literally gasp as she witnessed the transformation of my face. She remarked later that she had never seen anything like that transfiguration in her entire life. It must have looked amazing.

I have never doubted the intuitive process by which rebirthers and rebirthees come together. I can only reiterate my faith in the process by saying that not only did I get a rebirther who was willing to allow me the intimate experience of nursing, but she also had milk in her breasts from having given birth to her daughter, Kelly.

I was in ecstasy. It was for me the release of thirty-two years of deeply buried emotional upset. The end of a long search. I nursed only briefly. The experience itself was sufficient. Among the swirling mass of thoughts and feelings going on at that moment, one dominant feeling prevailed. An overwhelming sense of gratitude and love for Isara for knowing what to do and being willing to do it. Those two qualities I think mark the difference between mediocrity and excellence in rebirthing.

Claudia and Isara then helped me out of the tub and onto the nearby pad where I reclined and was covered with a large soft towel. I was still somewhat weak and helpless and it felt great. I wanted to be alone with my thoughts. Memories were starting to come in now and I wanted to be still and see the show. Both women understood this telepathically and said nothing. Sitting in silence, they touched my head and feet gently and waited.

I saw myself, my mother, the doctor and attendants in the delivery room. My perspective was from a point in the room about ten feet above the delivery table and slightly to the right of the doctor's shoulder.

The scene had the unreal quality of a science fiction movie. I watched myself emerging from the birth canal. I came out breathing and hungry and ready for life. I then saw the doctor present me to my mother who smiled and was proud. Noticing that I was hungry (I was making those same sucking sounds), the doctor offered me to my mother's arms and asked her if she wished to feed me right there. And here is where it all went South. I sensed a clear feeling of embarrassment in my mother, who after all had just endured the ignominy of lying for hours on a table with her legs spread wide apart while a group of masked strangers studied her gaping genitals. At this point, to bare her breasts and suckle her newborn child in front of all these people would just be too much to bear. Too high a confront. Simply more than her dignity could stand. She teetered a moment on the brink of re-consideration, then declined.

The shock of this rejection sent a jolt through my body. At that moment it was abundantly clear to my baby mind that I would go through life without even so much as a hope that I would ever get any nourishment from women in particular and people in general.

In a split second I saw with total clarity and perfect understanding why every single relationship I had had with a woman inevitably ended in incompletion. Dissatisfaction. Separation. I saw in that moment that not one love relationship I had ever had even had a prayer of being whole, complete or lasting. I was too busy working out my revenge. This made me very sad and I cried. Cried for all the lost love. Cried for all the broken hearts and unfulfilled hopes and aspirations. Cried for the subtle cruelties and perpetrations. My sadness was a sadness of remorse.

This soon passed and another, much lighter insight drifted by. I realized that on a visual and tactile level I, Gary, had been searching for the lost tit all my life. In that moment I was able to acknowledge my compelling lust for breasts. I loved them. Loved to look at them. Was irresistibly attracted to them. I even admitted to myself that when meeting a woman for the first time, I would inevitably look first at her breasts, then at her face or the rest of her body. I was obsessed. In fact for a while in my life I actually made many thousands of dollars photographing them for various mens' entertainment and nudist magazines. The thought even occured to me that I just might be living in Hawaii because there are more bra-less women per capita there than any other state in the country. Or maybe because people in Hawaii wear less clothing in general because of the climate. My imagination began to soar off into wild speculation at this point so I reined it in sharply.

More implications of this at-birth decision began to float in. I saw that, as life went on, I had generalized this thought of "no nourishment." It had affected my eating habits. I regularly ate and drank far more than I needed for good health. And I stuffed it down rapidly when I did eat. There never seemed to be enough. Even when I was "full," it was not the fullness of satisfaction. My generalization even included "not enough" money. No matter how much money I made, and at times I made quite a lot, it was never enough. I had smoked heavily for ten years before quitting, had been a compulsive gum chewer. It all fit. I had created my own personal nourishment shortage with a thought at birth, then had lived with it ever since. I was ready to give it up.

As if hearing that thought in their minds, Isara and Claudia both moved closer and began to love me up and give me nourishment. My whole body was one big pleasure-sensing neuron. They asked me if they could do anything for me. I was stunned. It somehow just hadn't occurred to me that I could ask a woman for what I wanted and get it, yet here were two friends waiting for me to tell them what I wished them to do for me. I was sure that I had been asked the question before, other times in other places, but I don't think I even heard it.

I love foot massages. The ladies gave me an exquisite foot massage that seemed to go on forever. Or was it that I was just experiencing total satisfaction every single moment and had lost my sense of time? Maybe that was the key. If I could experience total satisfaction each moment instead of worrying about an impending lack or shortage in the next, each moment would be full and I would experience fulfillment. Full-fill-ment! What a word! I love it.

I now forgive my mother for her unwillingness to nourish me when I was born.

I, Gary no longer need to get even with women for not giving me what I need.

Women are now happy to give me what I want and need.

The universe is filled with an infinite abundance of love, nourishment, money, sex and affection.

It is now OK for me, Gary, to ask for and receive whatever I need.

These were some of the affirmations I designed for myself after this first tub rebirth. I did them on tape, playing them back to myself at night and in a short time, the problems caused by this whole birth episode cleared up.

I really enjoyed writing these rebirth experiences for Sondra's book. It was part of my purpose in writing them to keep them light and amusing. Rebirthing is really and truly about having a good time and laughing while shoveling the shit out of the barn, you might say. Some of the most hilarious and silly good times I've ever had have been during rebirths, mine or others'. It is impossible for me to convey the value I've received from this truly divine process. I thank Leonard Orr for discovering it, Isara White for knowing what to do with it, and myself for having the courage and intuition to go and do it. Nothing has been the same since.

Well, all this has made me very hungry so I'm going out for a hot fudge sundae now, and while I eat it I'll write some affirmations and look at the *legs* of the pretty girls.

Gary Sohler

Rebirth Affirmations

1. I am breathing fully and freely.
2. I survived my birth, therefore my parents and doctor, and I myself, love life more than death and choose my survival.
3. My physical body is a pleasant and wonderful vehicle for my full and free self-expression.
4. I am glad to be out of the womb so I can express myself fully and freely.
5. I now receive assistance and cooperation from people.

6. I am safe, protected by Infinite Intelligence and Infinite Love, people and things no longer hurt me without my conscious permission.
7. I am no longer afraid of my breath.
8. I have the right and ability to express my hostility about my birth without losing people's love and support.
9. I am now willing to see my birth clearly.
10. Feeling all my emptiness won't destroy me.
11. I forgive myself for the pain I caused myself at birth.
12. Energy and vitality are my birthright.
13. My mother loves and appreciates me.
14. My mother is now glad that I was born.
15. My mother is now happy to get me out of the womb.
16. It was a privilege for my mother to have the honor to bring me into the world.
17. I am the way, the truth and the life. I came through her body and I am glad to be here. The entire universe is glad that I am here.
18. I no longer feel unwanted. The universe rejoices at my presence in it.
19. The universe is singing in my atoms.
20. My mother, father, family and friends are all glad that I was born and that I am alive.
21. Praise the Lord for the perfection of my living flesh.

Ten Practices of Theta Seminars and Rebirth International

1. Spiritual enlightenment; Being, Thought, Universe (Body)
2. Rebirthing
3. Unraveling the five biggies and the experience of loving
4. Affirmations and goals
5. Spiritual community
6. Prosperity consciousness
7. New age politics and ecology
8. Daily recreation and manual labor

9. Yoga exercises
10. Physical immortality

Ten Yoga Exercises Received from Babaji

1. 3 breathing cycles through mouth on toes
2. 3 breathing cycles through nose on toes
3. Head forward while holding breath
4. Head forward and to sides while holding breath
5. 3 breathing cycles through mouth on toes
6. Reclining feet together breathing—3, 5, or 7 times
7. 3, 5, or 7 sit-ups
8. Concentration while breathing—1 minute +
9. Concentration without breathing—15 seconds +
10. Chant OM or Abubabaji's mantras

Leonard Orr, founder of rebirthing, installed these practices in all rebirther trainings in Spring 1977, because they produce better mental and physical health and process the feelings activated by rebirthing, especially the feelings of hopelessness and helplessness surrounding birth.

Definitions of Rebirthing

The purpose of Rebirthing is to remember and re-experience birth. The experience begins a transformation of the subconscious impression of birth from one of primal pain to one of pleasure. Effects on life are immediate: as negative energy patterns held in the mind and body start to dissolve, "youthing" replaces aging, and life becomes more fun.

Rebirthing is:
1. The science of not holding your breath and rejuvenating your body with divine energy . . . Breaking a person out of un-

conscious holding patterns in regard to breathing.
2. Grease for the slide home.
3. A *scientific* pentecostal experience.
4. Baptism of the Holy Spirit with power.
5. Inflow of Divine Energy.
6. Re-learning to breathe.
7. A *physical* experience of Infinite Being.
8. A growth experience focused on releasing the trauma rather than re-experiencing it. (You can re-experience it a million times and get better at it.)
9. An energy release.
10. A cure for sub-ventilation using hyperventilation.
11. Learning to relax on a Cosmic Level.
12. Cleansing the mind and body of negative mental mass (tension).
13. A technique of spiritual healing.
14. Rebuilding the body with prenatal life energy.
15. Removing tension and blocks to full aliveness and health of human flesh.
16. Producing a perpetual state of health and bliss.
17. Renewal of divine nature in human form.
18. Regeneration of human perfection.
19. Dynamic energy.
20. Divine orgasm.
21. Release from mortal bondage.
22. Becoming aware of the energy that the body has always channeled.
23. Transubstantiation of the etheric vortices.
24. Letting go to the natural pulsation that's in the core of the organism.
25. Yielding to the metaphysical throb.
26. I didn't get high to die.
27. The practical mystical experience.
28. Pumping negative thought, feelings, and illness out of the body with the breath.
29. A breathing mantra.

Unexpurgated Definitions:
1. Masturbation of the mind.
2. Cosmic come.
3. Divine Infant shaking the shit out of the traumatized infant.

To learn more about rebirthing write or call:

Rebirth International   Inspiration University
c/o Rima Star   Campbell Hot Springs
6809 Daugherty   or   P.O. Box 234
Austin, TX   Sierraville, CA 96126
(512) 453-1724   (916) 994-8984 or
                                         (916) 994-3677

5 Spiritual Purification Practices For Conscious Breathers (from Babaji and Leonard Orr)

The purpose of Spiritual Purification is to purify the body, mind and emotions of negative thoughts and feelings. Without Spiritual Purification, Physical Immortality is a joke. The following are powerful purification practices. Don't let their simplicity fool you. Conscious breathers will benefit immeasurably by making these practices an integrated part of their day-to-day lives. They take nothing away from us (but our negativity). They give everything—including joy, bliss, happy relationships, prosperity consciousness and physical health. Read through the following list of practices and pick out the ones you are intuitively drawn to. Do only those that are pleasurable to you at this time.

All Spiritual Practices should be pleasurable, since pleasure is an aspect of love and love is the fundamental quality of the infinite.

1. *AIR.* Twenty connected breaths a day; also when in the midst of negativity or disturbing emotions. An hour of conscious connected breathing daily will energize the body and purify the mind.
2. *FIRE.* Watching a flame (such as a candle) or sitting close to a fire will clean the energy body. Putting ordinary food into the fire is the basis of the fire ceremony. Doing it in the forest has special value. (There is more about this in the next section.)

3. *WATER.* Bathing at least once a day while immersed in warm water. Doing twenty connected breaths or an hour of connected breathing multiplies the power of the water.
4. *EARTH.* Forming a conscious relationship to the planet will ground you and make your other purifications more beneficial to yourself and others. Manual labor and sports also act as a ground. Bathing in natural streams, lakes and oceans is very beneficial. Living in, or regularly visiting, a natural setting is a subtle yet powerful purification practice. Diet is important. Being a vegetarian, developing a preference for fruits, nuts, and natural foods, is helpful,
5. JAPA. It is one of the oldest methods of spiritual purification. Chanting or repeating silently to yourself the name(s) of God is a device to attune yourself to your own divinity. According to Babaji, *Om Namaha Shivaiva* is the oldest name for God. If this is not comfortable, use your own form. The idea is consciously to acknowledge your connection with Infinite Being and evoke your connection to God's presence with the continuous remembrance of God's name.
6. *FASTING.* Abstaining from food one day a week gives the body a rest and actually increases your enjoyment of food. Your body will gently guide you into longer fasts if this is what it desires.
7. *THOUGHT.* One of the two most powerful methods of spiritual purification. Improve the quality of your ideas and you will improve the quality of your life. You create your experience of life every moment whether you realize it or not. Examining your thoughts and changing the negatives into positives is a ludicrously simple, yet powerful, practice.
8. *UNCONDITIONAL LOVE, HUMAN RELATIONSHIPS.* As children we learned to disinherit whole aspects of ourselves in order to get mommy's and daddy's, our teacher's, our peers' and our society's approval. These denied parts float around in our consciousness searching to be readmitted to ourselves and demanding our attention. When you feel fragmented, or as if something inside of you is controlling you, it is one of these

denied parts of yourself seeking your love. You must love your monsters unconditionally. They are misplaced powers and when you take in your "prodigal sons," you will have more energy, more aliveness, more awareness and more love.

In terms of Spiritual Purification, Unconditional Love is a primary aspect of Infinite Being. By loving yourself unconditionally, you come closer to seeing yourself as your creator sees you. Love will actually move the molecules of your body. Together with creative thought, there is nothing that love cannot accomplish, nothing that cannot be transformed. All relationships embody our past conditioning, at least partially, until we are free of it.

Spiritual Purification makes one fit to live on the planet. "Heaven really is on earth, and those that don't realize this have to leave." Make these practices a fun part of your life. It is your choice to purify yourself or not. But if you don't, death will. Physical death is an involuntary method of spiritual purification.

Share these ideas with those you love and those you hate. Everyone deserves to be happy.

Fire Purification

The seven biggies of spiritual purification are: (1) OM NAMAHA SHIVAIYA, (2) Thinking, (3) Earth, (4) Water, (5) Air, (6) Fire, (7) Human Relationships—Love.

Fire is magical and mystical stuff. Without fire your body couldn't exist. The fire in your digestive system is what makes the food turn brown when it goes out the other end. You have fire in your blood and in every cell, as well as earth, water and air. A creative thought sends fire through your nervous system. Without fire your body would be ice.

If you watch fire you will notice that it flows just like water—only fire flows up and water flows down.

The purpose of fire purification is to clean your energy body. I've gotten into a routine of doing fire purification at least three times a week on Tuesdays, Thursdays and Saturdays. It seems to take at least four hours with a big fire, the flames of which sometimes go above my head, to produce a completed energy cycle. After I get a bed of coals and have some real nice flames covering the wood I do the basic fire ceremony which I learned from Babaji. (Some American Indian tribes do this same ceremony.) The ceremony is simple; it consists of throwing ordinary food into the fire while saying OM NAMAHA SHIVAIYA. The food which you offer into the fire can be grains, nuts, fruits, vegetables or whatever your favorite foods are. If you smoke you can even offer tobacco. If you have a problem with certain foods or cigarettes I would definitely offer these things into the fire each time you do fire purification.

When I put the offering in the fire I always experience a burst of white light in my aura and all my senses get sharper. I also notice that I have built a successful relationship with fire. It has become my friend. It is more intelligent than most people. It responds to my thoughts and speaks back to me. As an aspect of my being, fire cooperates with me and serves me. The fire ceremonies are an act of respect and somehow they have given me a certain power in my relationship to fire. I listen to fire and fire listens to me and obeys. Fire as a fundamental aspect of divine substance does work for me as God answers prayers. My personal fires never burn out of control because fire loves me. It is my friend. I have discovered some of the divine secrets of fire.

Because of my awareness of my energy body through conscious breathing I experienced the relationship of fire purification in the cleaning of my energy body the very first time, but it has taken several months of meditation in the presence of this wonderful friend to learn its secrets. We can only learn the secrets of fire from the fire itself, just as you can only learn the secrets of breathing from the breath itself. We learn the secrets of water by meditating in the water and the secrets of earth by meditating on it. Earth, air, water and fire are the eternal principles of the physical universe. To know them and to love them and to be known and loved by them is part of a conscious relationship to

God. If you spend enought time with fire, Babaji will speak to you through the fire the same way he spoke to Moses in the burning bush. He will give you his Name:

Fire purification is as much fun as conscious breathing and conscious bathing, as well as conscious eating or fasting. It also involves earth purification when you are cutting and carrying wood. Fire purification seems to be equal to and as powerful as earth, air and water purification. Fire purification produces profound energy changes in my mind and body that are as significant as rebirthing or fasting. Fire reaches different energies. For example, I've noticed that it burns away death-urge material and anger very efficiently. It also opens up subconscious material that can be dissolved by a long warm bath afterwards.

You can do fire purification on one level with a candle or in a fireplace. I enjoy doing most out in the forest. The most dramatic energy changes occur after three or four hours. When I've done enough I feel strong, calm, peaceful and my mind thinks clearly. I also feel physically tired and satisfied as a result of cutting all that wood with an axe. Fire purification is a wonderful experience of nature and the physical universe. You learn the ultimate secrets of fire from the fire itself. You just have to do it. You have to spend enough time with the fire to learn its secrets. In the city you can use a barbecue tray with charcoal and burn one or two pieces of wood at a time.

Fire is a powerful element. Whether using a candle, a fireplace, or out in the forest, it is important to practice adequate fire safety. With candles I recommend that you have a metal or glass dish the radius of which is as much as the height of the candle so that if the candle falls over it can't fall out of the dish. With a fireplace be sure that the logs can't roll out and that there is a proper screen to keep sparks from flying into the room and setting the house on fire. Without proper fire precautions you may get more fire purification than you expected! Fire purification takes more consciousness than water purification and some techniques of earth and air purification.

When in the forest I recommend that you take a shovel or a

around the fire 5 to 10 feet may be enough. If there is a wind it is important to build your fire in a deep fire pit 2 to 3 feet deep and clear the area around the fire of all hazardous material like pine needles within 200 feet. I recommend that you go to your local forest service ranger station and receive the basic lecture about fire prevention. Obviously you need a fire permit or permission from the land owner whenever you do fire purification on property you don't own.

Fire purification is a very great technique of self-evolution. It can clean and heal your energy body as well as your mind and physical body. Probably a very few American Indians are the only people in this country who really understand its mysteries. You can only learn these mysteries by being with the fire alone, with the purpose of meditating on the fire and your energy in God. In 1974, when I started teaching people the secrets of breathing, there was practically no one in the country who understood the mysteries of the breath. In 1982 there are one to two million people in the country who know how to contact the energy of God through breathing. Obviously it is my goal to spread the practice of fire purification as I have spread the practice of air purification. In addition to being good for you, it is also good for nature: it cleans up our forests and prevents forest fires.

It is amazing how simple and how powerful the true practices of aliveness are. Fire purification enables me to burn away the negative energies I absorb from groups. It clears the effects of being a leader. It makes my life more pleasurable. It burns away death-urge material very efficiently. It always turns anger into peace.

Consciousness Village/Campbell Hot Springs is loaded with the true riches of earth, air, water and fire. We have pure air, we have natural hot and cold running water, we have all kinds of terrain and we have an abundance of wood for fire and plenty of space for many people to do fire purification in solitude. You can practice all the seven biggies of spiritual purification here at Consciousness Village/CHS.

(For more information about fire and other methods of spiritual purification, please see my new book *Physical Immortality.* It is available by mailing $12 to Inspiration University, Box 234, Sierraville, CA 96126, or see your local bookstore.)

6 Physical Immortality

There is an alternative to physical death. Although we have all been heavily programmed to believe otherwise, it is possible to go on living forever without dropping the physical body. Physical immortality, perpetual longevity, eternal life in your living flesh, is now a practical possibility.

There is also an alternative to aging. The habit of affirming the power of death causes not only death but also many illnesses and states of weakness leading up to death.

The idea that death is inevitable has killed more people than all other causes of death combined.

The practice of physical death has been popular for a long time, and many people are determined to die and maintain the tradition. But the necessity of physical death is now being seriously questioned, and there is a growing body of literature (the "immortalist" literature) dedicated to overthrowing death's domination of man. Philosophers and scientists now suspect that death has been popular for so many centuries because no one ever questioned it. In the past, people have avoided the study of death because they were afraid it would happen to them.

Why study it now? It is true that there can be no scientific proof for physical immortality. The only possible proof would be to live forever, and who can measure forever? This chapter could be read only as an exercise for your mind, like a koan. From a practical standpoint, however, accepting the philosophy of physical immortality has at least as much value as having a deathist mentality. And it may be better for the health of your mind, body and spirit. The transformation from mortality to immortality is easier than you think.

Modern medical scientists are beginning to affirm that it is not only possible, but increasingly likely, that we can build a permanent health consciousness. This idea is dramatically supported by recent longevity statistics; the average life span has more than tripled in the last two centuries. It is expected to increase even more rapidly in the future. Predictions of people living two hundred, or even five hundred, years in perfect health and youthful appearance, are becoming more common. Some scientists are declaring that people eventually will be able to banish physical death, in the traditional sense, from human experience.

It is certain that there are people living on this earth who are more than two hundred years old, but who do not reveal their true ages because it is not generally safe to do so. Some people may be—undoubtedly are—much older than that. Consider that, having mastered the physical body, a person would function totally naturally in the physical environment, and so would look just like everyone else. In other words, an immortal body would look like any other body! Of course, immortal bodies would not be subject to traditional limitations; but only people whose minds are open and susceptible to the possibility could be aware of that.

The idea of physical immortality may sound new, but it has been around since literature began. Spiritual Masters of all religions have taught these ideas for centuries. In fact, it is quite possible that most of the great religious literature was inspired by the immortal Masters. The Siddha tradition in India embraces the idea that some people have been around since the human body evolved, waiting for the rest of us to catch on. But in our culture, you are unlikely to be exposed to the Siddhic view. You might have heard stories about those spiritual Masters who have conquered death, but they sounded like pleasant myths. And if you are personally loyal to the concept of death, the deathist philosophy, the deathist theology, the deathist psychology, then you probably never thought of investigating any other alternative. All religious literature has stories about longevity and immortality, but they have rarely been accepted as historical reality. The Bible tells us that Enoch, the father of Methusda, was the first man to conquer death. He lived thousands of years before Jesus. Elijah lived several centuries before Jesus and conquered death. *Jesus himself did not conquer death to prove he was better or different than we are, but to teach us that we can do it for ourselves.* Jesus died and arose from the dead because man still did not understand the message. He created his death and resurrection with auto-suggestion.

If you love your body as much as God loves your body, you could live forever. (If you notice that you are already resisting some of these ideas, it is because people generally don't like to have their beliefs attacked; if you have a particular idea about death, you will tend to resist any attempt to change it. In other words, some people resent an attack on their belief about death even if their belief is killing them!)

The Intelligence that created the physical universe created the human body out of the same substance. It follows that the human body, which contains the highest expression of that Intelligence, should last as long as the rest of the physical universe. Destroying the body by dying is an insult to the Intelligence that created it.

Winning the game of life by mastering your body is important; but ultimately it is impossible to lose. As long as you have a spirit, mind or body, each contains the other within itself. The soul will go on creating bodies until it is perfect. In this sense, physical immortality is inevitable for everyone. So why not practice the end from the beginning—and contain the alpha and omega of existential reality within yourself?

Most people believe that death is beyond their control. Some blame it on God. But if you believe that God controls death, then you make God a murderer. Finding that idea unpalatable, other people devised the idea of Satan and blamed death on him. Others blame death on Mother Nature. Regardless of where the blame is assigned, the idea is that there is someone or something out there in the universe that is going to kill you. It is impossible to walk around in a universe that is out to destroy your physical body without being nervous about it. If you carry in your mind the notion that the universe is a hostile place, don't be surprised if your spouse or your parents or your children act hostile. What they are actually doing is symbolically lashing out at God, who is supposedly planning on murdering them. Alan Harrington, in *The Immortalist,* says that humans have always hated God for putting them in a closed universe from which they cannot escape alive. Stanley Spears, in *Stop Dying and Live Forever,* has a beautiful phrase: "Death is a grave mistake."

Physical immortality can be defined as endless existence; specifically, the endless existence of your physical body in perpetual health and youthfulness. The goal, then, is to master the physical body. Your physical body is obviously your most valuable possession. Thomas Carlyle said, "There is but one temple in the Universe and that is the human body. Nothing is holier than that high form. We touch heaven when we lay our hand on the human body." People, however, will take better care of their houses and other possessions than they will of their physical body. Isn't it amazing that a contractor has the ability to construct a physical building that can last for hundreds of years and doesn't use the same ability to construct a lasting body? He doesn't take the same responsibility for his own body. Now if you have the power in your mind to construct an immortal building, then why don't you have the power to construct an immortal body?

The fact is that people allow their physical body to be destroyed easily, sometimes without a protest. The human body took millions of years to evolve, and it is truly a marvelous thing. Why would God want to destroy after seventy years something that took millions of years to evolve? It is an insult to let some tiny little organism or germ destroy it. The truth is that the same Infinite Intelligence that evolved your physical body knows what to do about micro-organisms and can protect your body from them. It can protect your body from other human beings. It can also protect you from Mother Nature, or Satan, or God, or whatever you *think* kills your physical body. Actually, it is your mind that creates the death of your body. *The truth is that all death is suicide.*

Some people say to us, "Well, I am willing to live forever if it doesn't get too bad." That is a complete cop-out. It only gets too bad if they have not given up their loyalty to death. In the traditional perspective, people think that you age, you get sick and you die. The truth is that you die, you get sick and you age. You create symptoms in your physical body that make it socially acceptable for you to leave it. A currently popular one is cancer.

Cancer is a conflict between your life urge and your death urge which manifests in the cells. The conflict will be resolved depending on your belief. If you constantly reaffirm that death is inevitable, then death is the result you will get. If you believe that cancer is curable, then that is the result you will get. Leonard has worked with people on their death urge, and they claim that he cleared up their terminal cases of cancer. Actually all he did was get them to change their concept of death, to give up the notion that death is inevitable, and also to deal with the specific consciousness factor from their family tradition that was contributing to the symptoms. *There is nothing that is incurable except that which you acknowledge as incurable. To change your body all you have to do is change your mind; your body will change automatically.*

Your beliefs obviously control your physical body. If you believe it is raining outside, you will probably put on a coat or a raincoat, or take an umbrella, whether or not it is actually raining. If you believe that it is, it will affect your behavior and what your body does. If you *believe* that you cannot bend your finger, you will never bend your finger. And if you believe that you can bend it, you will bend it.

You were conditioned by your parents and society to believe you were going to die around seventy; this is merely a belief system and it can be changed. *Remember that thought is creative; what the mind thinks, it produces.* This is the law of cause and effect. That is, thought causes everything that exists. And so what you think becomes very important. If you think you are going to die, you will. If you think you are going to be reincarnated, you will be reincarnated. If you think it, you make it true.

There is only one way that you can object to this truth and that is with thought; which only further proves that thought is creative. You create everything in your body with thought. You are "at cause" over your body. You are also at cause over death. Thought is creative *and* uncreative. What thought creates it can also uncreate.

Are you still having trouble accepting these concepts? Science offers further support for the possibility of physical immortality. The average life span in the Western world has doubled in the last two hundred years. It was thirty-five years in 1776, and in 1976 had reached seventy years. All the scientific measurements of technology indicate that our knowledge is doubling every ten years. If that is true, and the knowledge of longevity accelerates at the same rate, then the average age of our generation could be one hundred and fifty! By the time we get to be one hundred and fifty, we will have passed through another generation, which, if the life span doubles during that generation, will be three hundred. The United Nations has committees that are seriously planning population statistics based upon life spans of one hundred and fifty. People in our culture will be programmed into being immortal even without learning the concept, because there will be a quantum leap and everybody will be swept along.

When you start talking about the prospect of physical immortality, you have to postulate the rejuvenation of the body and even the reversing of the aging process. Leonard coined the word *youthing* which is the opposite of aging. A simple technique in developing a youthing attitude is to affirm on each birthday that you are one year younger. Follow it up all year by affirming that you are getting younger and more attractive. Affirm youthing for yourself and affirm all of its characteristics. If you don't succeed the first year, try again.

Your body has the ability to produce new cells. For example, when you cut yourself, your body builds brand new cells to repair the cut. Scientific theory tells us that the body totally renews itself every eleven months. If all of your cells die and are replenished every eleven months, then your body is never more than eleven months old! It is a paradox that the principle of death is what makes physical immortality possible. Death of the cells is one of the ways that death serves physical immortality. Your body is a constantly flowing stream of life. The cells are constantly changing and the fact is that your mind is the only element that "ages." The mind "creates" older new cells that correspond to the beliefs programmed into it. Earl Nightingale says that a man's face after forty is his own fault, and what his face looks like depends upon what he spends his evenings thinking about. It is very true that thoughts of fear, pain and grief create ugliness and old age. By affirming youthing instead of aging, you can control the "age" of your own being!

Isn't it amazing that babies always come out the same age? It does not matter whether the mother is sixteen or forty-six, the babies always come out the same age. The baby, the new being, is created as a part of the woman's body, regardless of her age. It illustrates that you have as much youth potential in your body as anybody.

We have several alternatives when it comes to producing cells:

1. Cells reproduce themselves exactly the same as they were.
2. Cells reproduce themselves worse.
3. Cells reproduce themselves better.
4. Cells don't reproduce themselves.
5. New cells are produced that you never had before.

If you are producing a scab or scar tissue, then you are producing cells that turn out worse than the original ones. If you are losing weight then you are not reproducing cells. If you are gaining weight then you are producing new cells. Our mind controls which alternative works and which set of cells and part of our body is affected. Consider the possibilities you have in controlling the cells you reproduce: you can flow your stream of life in either direction, youthing or aging. You might want to youth for ten or twenty years and stay there for a few decades, or maybe a century or two. Then you might want to try aging again. These are actual realistic possibilities and the spiritual Masters have demonstrated all of these for us. In fact, the Masters who have evolved themselves to the point of dematerializing and rematerializing the whole body at will, can concentrate and transform their body into that of a female or a male, a child or elderly person. One of the most popular pieces of literature describing this ability is *Autobiography of a Yogi* by Yogananda, in which there are all kinds of stories about Masters at that level. An even better source than that is *Life and Teachings of the Masters of the Far East.* Comprised of five volumes, it is the story of eleven American scientists and scholars who studied and lived with the Masters for three and one-half years in the 1890s. They had lived with the Masters for a year before they realized that the Masters had been materializing their food!

Even if death is inevitable, it won't hurt you to believe in physical immortality. It is the safest belief there is. If you are going to die anyway, the idea of physical immortality won't make a difference. So you might as well believe in it; it might have the practical benefits of making you feel healthy and wonderful while you are here. When you give up your mortal mentality, you will feel a wonderful difference.

You might say, "Yes, but these high hopes are really just reserved for those spiritual Masters." Today everyone is becoming a spiritual Master and, the fact is, you already are one. If you have the ability to destroy your physical body (which takes a whole lot of effort), you can just as well preserve your physical body, which is a whole lot easier. However, if you believe that death is inevitable, then you are in the process of dying right now.

Or you might say, "A hundred years is all I can take." That statement springs from a deep-rooted belief in suffering and limitation. You then have not yet experienced the fullness of health, joy, wisdom, peace and love. As you study this whole book carefully, you will discover that with it you are given the means to having these substantive qualities of life itself. And once you have them and life becomes deliciously wonderful, why leave?

John 3:16, the golden text of Christianity, says:

> For God so loved the world
> that He gave His only begotten
> Son that whosoever believeth in Him
> shall have everlasting life.

Leonard likes to point out that God evidently loves the world more than He loves Christians, because the world is still around and most Christians are either dead or looking forward to dying. The truth is that if you love your body as much as God does it will last as long as the physical universe. Somehow, Christians have misinterpreted John 3:16. It says that if you believe in the Son you will not perish but have everlasting life. Jesus said, "If any man keep my word, he shall never see death." The word is: "No man can take my life from me. I lay it down of myself and I take it again myself." When he saw that no one understood what he was telling them, Jesus decided to prove to humankind that death has no power. He predicted his death, and he predicted his resurrection. Then, by suggesting (or affirming) to himself what was his purpose, he did exactly as he said he would. Jesus created his death and resurrection by autosuggestion, and people still did not get the message.

Jesus took his body with him. He took total responsibility for his body and until we can be that responsible for our bodies we have no business comparing ourselves to Jesus. It is a goal to become like him however. Abubabaji, the Master we met in India, has a very personal friendship with Jesus. Through him we are gaining a new kind of love and respect for Jesus. He has said to us that if he told us what he knows about Jesus and his whereabouts right now we would not be able to move from our chairs.

The Bible presents death as the last enemy to be destroyed. The reason it is the last enemy is because it is the ultimate enemy. If you conquer death, you have time to conquer every other enemy. You have the time to deal with and conquer all enemies. The Bible calls death an enemy and the purpose of the whole Bible, according to the Genesis story, is to restore what Adam and Eve lost when they ate of the fruit of the tree of knowledge of good and evil. The promise was that they would be redeemed. The whole purpose of the Bible is to explain the redemption of the body.

How was death invented in the first place? People simply forgot how their minds work. They came to think of their bodies as being out of their control. When they injured their body they were unable to heal it; something "outside" seemed necessary. And aging developed when people forgot that they caused their own circumstances; they created worry, tension and fear to explain aging. Once the two syndromes of injury and aging were invented, parents passed them on to their children to justify themselves, and thereby developed a whole philosophy about weakness and death.

Kids get the idea that death is beyond their control. This idea is organically connected to sacrificing your divinity. As soon as parents convince their children that they don't have the right to run their own lives, death starts. Death of the body is just a natural result of death of the soul. As soon as you, for example, gave up your initiative and accepted that life is beyond your control, and is in fact controlled by somebody else, God became a projection of your parents. Your parents let you know that if you criticized them or hated them they would beat the hell out of you. You were taught, or you assumed, that God would do the same thing. If you would tell God he was a dirty rotten so-and-so for murdering people, then he would beat the hell out of you. And His beatings would last. They might be fatal. So nobody dared to tell God to go to hell.

The correlary of death is sickness. You must have an excuse to die, and if old age doesn't work then you have to have some other reason.

Lets go back to Genesis:

> Now the serpent was more subtle than
> any beast of the field which the Lord
> God had made. And he said unto the
> woman: Yea, hath God said, Ye shall
> not eat of any tree of the garden?

Implicit in that question is, first of all, the denial that she is God. The serpent said that God sets up the rules of the garden, not you;

therefore God is outside yourself. When Eve agreed to this, she denied her divinity. She was finished before she ate.

> And the woman said unto the serpent:
> we may eat of the fruit of the trees of
> the garden: but of the fruit of the tree
> which is in the midst of the garden,
> God hath said: "Ye shall not eat of it,
> neither shall ye touch it, lest ye die."

There are two trees in the middle of the garden, the tree of life and the tree of the knowledge of good and evil.

> And out of the ground made the Lord God
> to grow every tree that is pleasant to
> the sight, and good for food; the tree
> of life also in the midst of the garden,
> and the tree of the knowledge of good and
> evil.

The serpent directed Eve's attention to the tree of the knowledge of good and evil and Eve forgot about the tree of life. That is exactly what people have been doing for thousands of years. Our attention has been occupied by the tree of the knowledge of death. We have forgotten about the knowledge of life. If you eat of the knowledge of death, then you take it into your system and it becomes you. The reason that people could never figure out what kind of fruit the tree of the knowledge of good and evil was, was because they didn't read the statement. It says the tree of *knowledge*. Now what is the tree of knowledge? It is a body of knowledge. The belief that death is inevitable is that body of knowledge. To eat of the knowledge that death is inevitable automatically produces death.

> And the serpent said unto the woman:
> Ye shall not surely die; for God
> doth know that in the day ye eat
> thereof, then your eyes shall be
> opened, and ye shall be as God,
> knowing good and evil.

Again, the assumption is that she is not God. If she is tempted by that little idea, then she has already lost the battle. So if you are tempted by the idea that you are not God and therefore cannot determine the consequences of your own actions, then it is all over. When the Bible says that the serpent is subtle and crafty, you have to see that actually it is the preachers that are the subtle and crafty ones. They have taught you that you are not God and that you are a sinner. In order to sustain their position they have to lie about their position. Jesus said to the religious leaders of his day. "You are the children of the devil. You are liars and you are the children of the Father of all lies and the Father of all lies is that you are not God."

Once you have bought this interpretation, you have to produce an infinite amount of lies in order to support your own position ("I can't heal myself"; "I am weak"; "I don't have any power"; "I can't love"; etc.)

The original sin, thinking you are not God, is the sin which takes you out of heaven, because it makes you greater than God. In order to NOT be God, you have to have power to exempt yourself from his presence. To do this you have to think you are better than God. Therefore the paradox is that to admit that you are God is a source of humility.

What kills people? Well, some people are said to die by drowning, and yet there are yogi Masters who stay submerged for days or weeks without air and come out unharmed. We say that falling from heights kills people. What height is high enough? One person dies by falling off a step, another person might die by falling off a roof. In *From Here to Greater Happiness,* there is a story of two drunks who fell out of a four-story window and walked away unharmed because they didn't know they fell out. Then there is the Lufthansa stewardess who fell forty-five thousand feet out of an exploding airplane and lived through it. There are other incidents of people falling out of airplanes and landing in a plowed field and surviving. Some people fall off a small step ladder and die. So what height is high enough? So what is the appropriate height to kill people? If a person's unconscious death urge is strong enough, he can trip over the carpet and die.

There isn't any direct correlation between falling from heights and death. There isn't any direct correlation between any kind of disease and death, because there are incidences of curing everything. Death is the result of ignorance of cause. *Death is the result of holding the thought that death is inevitable.*

The Alternatives to Immortality

Most people believe there is only one answer to the question of mortality and immortality, and that whatever it is happens to everybody whether they believe it or not. Orthodox Christians believe that people die and go to heaven or hell, whether they like it or not. The reincarnationists believe that people die and are reincarnated, whether they like it or not. The atheists believe there is nothing after death, that death is the end, and that the Christians and reincarnationists are just deluding themselves.

Out of the three alternatives—physical death, physical immortality or dematerialization—the most popular alternative is physical death. There are all kinds of postulations about what happens after physical death:

1. The first one is nothing, or *annihilation.* Death is the end, and your mind and soul and body are totally destroyed or dissolved. Your individual consciousness ceases to exist altogether.

2. The second is entering the *astral world.* The astral world is a place where living forms are at a different rate of vibration than we now experience in the physical world. In the astral world, there is a whole scale of existence, ranging from unpleasant to pleasant. Unpleasant is popularly referred to as hell; and pleasant is popularly referred to as heaven. (If you are Catholic, the middle ground is purgatory, which is sometimes pleasant and sometimes not.) The astral world is really a world of the mind in which you are adding more and more thought and more and more ideas to the original concept until it finally materializes and takes on a reality of its own.

Since the astral world is the world of the mind, you don't have to go anywhere to get into the astral world. And that leads to the conclusion that the value of the death process is highly overrated. Physical death is highly overrated because all it does is destroy the physical body. If you are miserable in the physical body, experiencing the death process to reach the astral world won't change anything. You are not going to a higher place; there is no higher place. The whole of reality is right where you are, where you create it. And if you can't find it right where you are in your present physical body, destroying your physical body won't help you one bit. Dying is not going to work as a way out. *The only thing that will move you to a higher "place" is the quality of your thoughts!* Heaven is not a place, it is the experience of divine love.

3. Another alternative is *reincarnation.* People think that to reincarnate you die and come back through the womb again. But you do not have to go through physical death in order to reincarnate, because reincarnation can be accomplished through the reincarnation of your mind. You can reincarnate without going through physical death by changing the concepts your physical body is embodying. You can go through a total transformation of your physical body just by changing your concepts! Also, with reincarnation through the womb, the chances are that the body you come out with, after you go through death and come back, will be similar to what you have now anyway. Creating a belief system that includes reincarnation does not necessarily change the mental programming that created you in the first place, because the mind carves the body. So the value of going through the birth-death cycle is highly overrated.

4. Another alternative is *sleep,* or suspended animation. It is the idea that you enter into a state of unconsciousness until, as some Christian groups believe, you resume consciousness at the Second Coming of Christ. (Some reincarnationists believe that you are unconscious until you reenter the body.)

5. Another alternative is *resurrection.* There are many modern cases of resurrection. Leonard has a newspaper clipping about a boy who was struck by lightning, which fused a chain of metal around his neck and also fused the zipper on his pants and put a great big hole in his baseball cap. He was playing baseball in a thunder storm and the lightning passed through his right heel,

burning a hole in his shoe. He was killed. He was dead for quite some time. But he came back to life, and the only damage to his body was to his heel, which healed. There are stories of medical students who studied anatomy by digging up graves to examine the cadavers. They recorded finding many coffins clawed up where people had tried to crawl out. Occasionally people crawled out of graves because the grave diggers were lazy and would bury them right under the surface. Morticians, doctors and preachers would get very upset when someone who had been in the grave for a week would crawl out and come walking down the street. That supposedly invalidated Christianity. The preachers didn't like that because if the ordinary person, who admits he is a sinner, could stay in the grave longer than Jesus and then come out, what was the purpose of believing in Jesus? It happened commonly enough so that the preachers, doctors, and morticians got together and passed legislation requiring burial six feet under. That made it really difficult to crawl out! As a result of moving graveyards and discovering caskets that were clawed upon inside, the undertakers decided it would be more humane to embalm people so they would not be resurrected to acute claustrophobia. Those of us who were raised in the age of embalming and burying people six feet under, don't even know about those stories. But esoteric books in dusty libraries carry these actual records. Or read the book, *Romeo Error.*

6. Another alternative is *possession.* Here there is a tremendous spectrum: Everything from *The Exorcist* to the *Seth Material,* which describes temporary possession (somebody possessing another person's body temporarily in order to fulfill their frustrated desires to be a teacher). The interesting thing about the possession literature is that some of them are generous enough to point out that if you sense your own spirit, thought, and reality yourself, then you don't have to be possessed by anybody in order to get higher wisdom, because you are already connected to it. In other words, your mind is immersed in Infinite Intelligence and if you just draw on it, you don't have to have any intermediary to deliver divine wisdom, so the authority of messages from spirits isn't any more valuable than that which you

can create in your own imagination. Just because a spirit doesn't have a body, that does not make him any smarter.

7. Another alternative would be to have the ability of *rematerialization.* That means to rematerialize the body without going through the womb. (A modern way to do this is to make a body in the laboratory, through the principle of cloning, which is now a realistic possibility.)

Most religions have presented their alternative as the only possibility and feel that everybody has to go through their alternative whether they like it or not. The alternative that we are presenting here is of *physical immortality,* which is the idea of keeping your physical body around forever. This has to include the ability to transform your body, as well as to bring about youthing as easily as aging. But it is important for us to acknowledge that if you want to die, that is perfectly OK. We think it is essential for you to know, however, that death is within your control and that you can do anything you desire about it. You have the choice.

We would like to conclude this discussion of physical immortality with one of the affirmations that Leonard invented, which will give your mind something to work with. The affirmation is:

> I am alive now, therefore my life urges are stronger than my death urges. As long as I continue to strengthen my life urges and weaken my death urges, I will go on living in increasing health and youthfulness.

That you are alive now is indisputable. Therefore your life urges are stronger than your death urges. Obviously, if your death urges were stronger than your life urges, you'd be dead! If your life urges have been strong enough to keep you alive up to this point, and you strengthen them, then they will keep you alive during the next moment. If they keep you alive in the next moment and you continue to strengthen them, they can keep you alive in every successive moment forever. If you keep weakening your death urges, they will not be strong enough to kill you in the future. If you go on living, and live with less death in your soul, then you are increasing your aliveness and your aliveness will be reflected in your physical body, which will have the appearance of vitality, youthfulness and health.

The ultimate accomplishment is to be able to dematerialize and rematerialize your body at will. If you can do that, you can do all the rest of them and utilize whatever alternative suits you. (The only alternative that is exclusive of all the rest is annihilation. If you use that one, anticipate its being permanent!)

Try working with Leonard's affirmation and with those that follow. You have nothing to lose but your death urge!

GENERAL ALIVENESS AND ENRICHMENT AFFIRMATIONS

1. My mind is centered in Infinite Intelligence that knows my good; I am one with the creative power that is materializing all my desires.
2. All the cells of my body are daily bathed in the perfection of my divine being.
3. I now have enough time, energy, wisdom and money to accomplish all of my desires.
4. I am always in the right place at the right time, successfully engaged in the right activity.
5. I now receive assistance and cooperation from people.
6. My days are filled with mental and physical pleasures.
7. I now give and receive love freely.
8. The more I win, the better I feel about letting others win; the better I feel about letting others win, the more I win; therefore I win all the time.
9. I daily make valuable contributions to the aliveness of myself, of others, and of humanity.
10. I no longer have to ask permission to do the things that I know should be done.
11. I now feel exhilarated and wonderful all of the time!
12. I do not have to suffer to get happiness.

13. My goodness keeps hanging around. Just because something is good, it does not mean that it has to go away.
14. All good things never end, they just keep getting richer.
15. I now enjoy accepting the good so that I can get more.
16. The more satisfied I become with the present situation, the more satisfaction I obtain.
17. I now feel sweet, joyous peace.
18. I have the right to indulge in laziness as long as it is pleasurable.
19. I am an ever-flowing spring of aliveness.

YOUTHING

1. I am alive now, therefore my life urges are stronger than my death urges; as long as I continue strengthening my life urges and weakening my death urges, I will go on living in health and youthfulness.
2. Life is eternal, I am life, my mind is the thinking quality of life itself and is eternal; my physical body is also eternal, therefore my living flesh has a natural tendency to live forever in perfect health and youthfulness.
3. My physical body is a safe and pleasurable place for me to be; the entire universe exists for the purpose of supporting my physical body and providing a pleasurable place for me to express myself.
4. All the cells of my body are daily bathed in the perfection of my divine being.
5. I am commissioned by the Infinite One (or God) to assist in the scheme of creation.
6. I am cooperating in the evolution of life, and in so doing my soul and body and their infinite possibilities are progressing in proportion to my desire to use all my powers and possibilities in spirit and in truth.
7. My physical organism is my natural universe, over which I alone will rule. It is my material cloak, or garment, through

which I will manifest the powers of divine nature. It is my fundamental servant.

8. I am progressing rapidly toward the conscious subjugation of matter and the complete lordship over all basic elements of life, which exist only by my permission as peaceful and obedient servants.
9. All the cells, tissues, and organs in my body are now youthing according to my desires.
10. The divine alchemist within is transforming the appearance of my body to express its eternal youthfulness.
11. My body is youthing; it daily expresses more health and strength.
12. I am now starting the youthing process; each birthday I will become a year younger.
13. I have eternal life—my body totally renews itself as long as I like.
14. I am cooperating in the progressive evolution of creation; the entire universe supports and assists my life and goals. My soul and body, with their infinite possibilities, are progressing in accordance with my desires. I now use all of my powers and possibilities in spirit and in truth.
15. My physical body is my most valuable possession.
16. The more I am good to myself, the more I enrich my aliveness.
17. I do not give my body a chance to self-destruct.
18. Each one of my cells grows in perfect youth, becoming more alive and energetic every day. Each cell replaces itself with a finer, purer, more perfect cell.
19. The only germs that can harm me are the germs of bad ideas.
20. My body is not one with pain; I can therefore let go of pain anytime I want.
21. My body is my loving servant; it is trying to teach me to give up false ideas so I can enjoy eternal life and all its pleasures.
22. As God, I have the ability to substitute health for sickness.
23. The more I am good to myself, the more I enrich my own aliveness.

HEALTH AND BODY CONSCIOUSNESS

1. I now feel exhilarated and wonderful all the time.
2. My skin is becoming beautiful and my oil glands function perfectly. In fact, my skin is getting younger.
3. Infinite Intelligence is healing my body.
4. My mother and my lovers now like my body.
5. My body is highly pleasing to (men) (women).
6. The purpose of my bloodstream is to clean out my whole body and keep it in perfect health.
7. I don't have to have a headache to make _____ _____ wrong.
8. Tension is no longer a problem of mine.
9. I am now willing to drop my tensions and feelings of helplessness and live in the glory of my natural divinity.
10. I have the right and ability to live without tension; I am loved by all.
11. I like myself even though I am tense, therefore I have no need to be tense.
12. My body will function perfectly with any amount of sleep.
13. I no longer need pains to get attention.
14. My perfect weight is _____ and all cells in excess will be washed out by my bloodstream.
15. My body is my servant which is getting me my perfect weight.
16. I am filling my life with pleasure to experience out pain.
17. My body is now bathed in the perfection of my Divine Being.
18. I rejoice in God's healing power in my body.
19. My body is not one with the pain, therefore I can let go of the pain anytime I want to.
20. My body is a loving servant which is trying to teach me to give up my false ideas so I can enjoy eternal life and all its pleasures.
21. Perfect vitality is the ground of my being and is manifesting in my physical body.
22. The Intelligence of pure spirit is expanding its perfect order in my mind and my body.

23. As God, I have the ability to substitute health for sickness.
24. My mind is thoroughly permeated with the recognition of its own life-giving power and thus does the work of substituting health for sickness.
25. My mind is tuned into the mind of _____, and therefore I can assist in healing _____. That perfection is being communicated to both of us, and enriches us.

* * * * * *

Babaji, Immortal Yogi Master
Shri Shri 1008 Shri Herakhan Wale Baba
P.O. Herakhan Mahadham, Via Kathgodam District
Nainital (U.P.), Pin Code 263126, India

7 Conscious Breathing for Airline Personnel Passengers and Other Advanced Beings

Why do I put airline personnel in a class with advanced human beings? The French have a saying, "Travel makes people grow younger." This saying was invented long before airplanes. Travel makes people more intelligent as well as younger.

I'm sure that when all the studies are completed, the long-term effects of travel, and flying especially, will reveal surprisingly beneficial effects on the mental and physical health of airline personnel. Flying is a profound self-improvement experience. It is possible to lose touch with the amazing phenomenon of a 747 taking off when you do it several times a day, but still difficult.

Although as a passenger for the past five years I have flown across the country approximately once a month and around the world at least once a year, I usually get awe-struck at least once during a flight. It may be the thought of this house on wheels leaving the ground. It might be the experience of looking down on the clouds, the realization of flying higher than the birds, or the "theoretical" knowledge of what the outside temperatures are at 35,000 feet.

My mind is expanded each time I look out the window and see the whole airport that this huge 747 is supposed to land in perceived in a few square inches of the window. When I am walking into the plane at the airport, I wonder how I can get the whole giant airport containing many planes back into that little window. Each plane is like a womb substitute, which actually helps unravel the birth-death cycle. The full implications of this are worth thinking about. I'm approaching this subject from the premise that all symptoms are actually healings in progress. The spirit, mind, and body of humans has the potential to heal anything and everything spontaneously and effortlessly. A little self-analysis of the emotional causation of the symptoms, letting go of negative thoughts, and a little conscious connected breathing can heal almost any human condition, mental or physical, and restore health and bliss. The realization that all undesirable sicknesses are temporary is a wonderful thought when you are in the middle of one.

I have thought for several years of writing this for airline personnel since doing voluminous research into breathing. I was finally motivated to put it on paper by a conversation with flight attendants at Chicago's O'Hare while between planes in December 1980. One flight attendant was on involuntary leave because of symptoms that were called epilepsy, nervous disorder, and many other things, but finally just tension. Her condition could most accurately be labeled *hyperventilation* or a *psychophysical rebirth.*

Some airline personnel have many negative thoughts and beliefs about flying. They think of flying as harmful to health for the following reasons:

1. Irregular sleep and work schedules produce stress on mind and body.
2. Changes in altitude, temperature and climate produce stress on mind and body.
3. Poor food and too much alcohol is a common problem among airline personnel.
4. Poor air, as a result of recirculating cabin air with too small a percentage of fresh air, is also a problem.
5. There is excessive exposure to cosmic radiation as a result of high altitudes.

6. Airline personnel constantly process the tensions, fears, negative emotions and bad vibrations of passengers in the compressed psychic atmosphere of the airplane cabin. It's like being trapped in the womb again, but with too much company—a psychic pollution of the energy body.

All of the items listed can be viewed as harmful—or as stimuli that produce advanced and superior people. Your conclusion is ultimately a belief that is subject to choice. It is up to you to decide whether flying is helpful or harmful to human health. Some people are healthier mentally and physically as a result of their flying experience, others are not.

I have talked with hundreds, perhaps thousands of airline personnel, mostly flight attendants and pilots who are students of the conscious breathing practice I started teaching in 1974. These people are among approximately half a million students who have reaped the benefits of conscious breathing during the past six years.

The conscious breathing method has also been called "rebirthing" because any conscious breathing stimulates birth memories for the obvious reason that birth is the moment of the first breath. If you study your own breathing rhythms for very long you will eventually remember the first breath and whether or not it was surrounded by what has popularly come to be known as "birth trauma." The truth is I have never met a person with a navel who wasn't suffering from some form of effects from birth trauma even though it might only be difficulty in getting out of bed.

Therefore, airplanes especially, but also automobiles, spontaneously stimulate emotional and physical symptoms that can be analyzed as the symbolic reliving of birth experiences.

Hyperventilation Syndrome

The explanation of these "nervous disorder" symptoms and many other phenomena common among airline personnel is very simple to myself and others who have done adequate research into this area. The best source of information comes from people who have figured out the nature of the "hyperventilation syndrome." The best information about hyperventilation comes from researchers who have experimented with it personally. I have thousands of students who have done hundreds of voluntary hyperventilation sessions. Hundreds of my students are medical doctors who have each done dozens or hundreds of personal hyperventilation sessions in the process of learning breath mastery.

The truth is that hyperventilation is only possible in people who are habitually underbreathers. What is not known, particularly in the Western world, is that perhaps over 90 percent of all people are underachievers of breath. The three main reasons for this are:

(1) The Western style of birth trauma
(2) Negative habits of thought
(3) The conveniences of civilization: the fact that most people walk so little and do so little manual labor, both of which would stimulate breathing. For all practical purposes we may say that everyone is susceptible to hyperventilation.

In fact, after teaching conscious breathing to over a half million people and training thousands of successful professional breathing teachers, I have concluded that people who have had personal experiences of hyperventilation voluntarily, or even involuntarily, are better off than they realize. However, involuntary hyperventilation experiences, especially, are usually fearful and upsetting for people.

Hyperventilation is the Breath of Life attempting dramatically to free itself from a lifetime of unconscious neglect. Although an involuntary hyperventilation "attack" seems to be triggered by a tense situation, a deeper look reveals that people who hyperventilate spontaneously have lived in a context of safety and security. Hyperventilation may be a disease of the well-off psychologically. What I've noticed in my hundreds of thousands of students when I looked for a common denominator is that they feel safe in their own minds (at least safe enough to consciously investigate the source of their own fears and anxieties rather than to run from them into popular methods of escape). Most of my students are functioning fairly successfully, are adventurous, willing to experiment with life, and operate from their own authority. They are responsible for themselves mentally, spiritually and physically.

Hyperventilation is your spirit, your personal aliveness, your breath busting out of its prison—a tense, over-active life. The human breath is the most powerful healing power in the mind and body. The simple act of daily breathing is the ultimate healer, but it is neglected, taken for granted, and inhibited. The science of breathing has been taught for thousands of years in India, but Westerners are perhaps more ignorant about breathing than any other ordinary activity. Think about it!

Mass Hyperventilation

A small-town, midwestern elementary school news item illustrates most of my points. One morning a boy fainted during choir practice. Several other children in the auditorium where they were singing fainted also, or were overtaken by convulsions or hysterical behavior such as excessive sobbing or fear. This hyperventilation-like behavior spread instantaneously throughout the school until over 100 of the 400 children were involved. The "epidemic" eexcitement lasted for about four hours. The children were all sent to the local hospital for checkups and all were released after a few minutes. They had all recovered completely by the time they reached the hospital and were feeling great except for coping with all the anxious and worried adults around them.

No mention of hyperventilation was made by the local school or medical authorities because they were totally ignorant of the literature on the subject. It was only mentioned later by outside consultants brought in to help explain the mysterious epidemic.

One thing was mentioned in the news story that probably even the medical consultants couldn't explain, yet the phenomenon is well-known to myself and my fellow researchers. The whole school was evacuated during this incident and a strange odor was reported to have filled the whole school building. The fire department was called in to investigate the possibility of gas leaks or even a gas bomb. Nothing was found. I believe the odor was what I call the "anesthesia" phenomenon. As a result of an extensive follow-up investigation of a few hundred thousand hyperventilation experiences, we have found that fainting normally occurs only in people who have been anesthetised during their lives. The theory is that rapid breathing literally pumps the anesthesia stored in the body out of the body on the exhale and has the same effect on the way out of the body through the breathing mechanism as it did on the way in. Scientific observers can actually smell ether in the room coming off the exhale and the person breathing can taste it.

This theory has been validated by hundreds of medical observers informally over the past four years. Formal research projects are presently being done on this phenomenon at universities.

The following is a list of symptoms that are associated with the hyperventilation syndrome:

- Rapid breathing
- Forced or heavy breathing
- Involuntary breathing
- Difficulty breathing including ashtma attacks
- Tingling or vibrating sensations in hands or feet
- Choking
- Tetany (a medical term for temporary paralysis or cramps)
- Light-headedness or dizziness
- Hysterical crying
- Irrational feelings of fear or terror
- Fainting
- Out-of-body experiences
- Temporary insanity
- Localized feelings of extreme pressure on body parts
- Strong energy flows
- Fluctuating body temperature

- Extreme sweating or inconsolable cold
- Confusion
- Claustrophobia
- Headache
- Body rushes
- Full-body orgasmic feelings
- Spiritual or religious visions
- Dramatic Telepathic experiences
- Nausea
- Dryness of mouth
- Buzzing or ringing in the ears
- Birth memories or dream-like states
- Euphoria and blissful states
- Color fantasies and vivid color perception
- Muscle spasms including epileptic-type seizures
- Death and resurrection experiences

Most of the above symptoms are explainable in terms of the release of suppressed primal psycho-physical memories. For example, tetany can be explained as releasing suppressed tensions accumulated and stored in the brain during infancy. The paralysis observably pulls the body into fetal poses during its most intense moments. Excessive sadness can usually be correlated to the unlimited sadness that infants sometimes experience during birth or early infancy. Fear is usually traced to memories of feelings during contractions at birth, the actual expulsion, and early separation from mother.

All of these states are symptoms that occur and disappear after a few minutes of continued breathing. The symptoms are caused by past thoughts and feelings. A symptom is the manifestation of an old negative thought in your body so that you can release it through your breath. All symptoms are healings in progress: either the spirit and mind are healing the body, or the spirit and body are healing the mind. But breathing is an ultimate healer. It can heal anything.

Thinking, breathing, touching, simple exercises and loving ser-
vice can and do heal everything. That is, changing your thoughts,
learning to breathe intuitively, and receiving frequent massages or
body work have healed every kind of illness known to man.
During an average conscious breathing session, people don't experience all of the above symptoms. But people usually have one
or more of them, sometimes only the pleasurable ones. The symptom is rarely painful. In fact, most people think of this dramatic
psycho-physical memory phenomena as interesting or even fun.
The symptom is a real body sensation, but continued breathing
rhythm causes it to disappear in a few minutes. Your breath and
spirit releases the symptom from your mind and body and you feel
free and clean. Once you have experienced your ability to breathe
away symptoms during a conscious breathing session, you can use
this ability to heal almost any form of mental and physical sickness. Breathing doesn't cause the symptom, relaxation does, by
permitting a negative thought to manifest, then more breathing
and relaxation dissolves the symptom and its cause—a thought.
Conscious breathing is not hyperventilation. It is a relaxed
breathing rhythm. However, a certain percentage of students do
experience hyperventilation symptoms during some of their early
sessions, or when they neglect their breathing. When conscious
breathing is done daily like eating, it maintains a healthier balance
in the blood as well as the energy body.

What is Conscious Breathing?

Conscious breathing is a physical, mental and spiritual experience, but mostly physical and spiritual. Feelings are usually rich
and intense, but rational thought is often "bypassed."
The physical part consists of connecting your inhale to your exhale in a relaxed rhythm. To connect your inhale to your exhale
means to merge them so that your breathing feels and sounds like

an unbroken circle. Relaxed breathing means that your inhales and exhales are complete and full, but not forced. Your breathing should not be too fast nor too slow. The rhythm of breathing is done mostly through the nose, but it is okay to breath through the mouth occasionally. Conscious breathing is done mostly in the chest, with emphasis on breathing with the lungs instead of the diaphragm or belly.

The spiritual dimension of conscious breathing is the heart of the matter. The purpose of conscious breathing is not primarily the movement of air, but the movement of energy. If you do a relaxed connected breathing rhythm for more than a few minutes, you will experience dynamic energy flows in your body. These energy flows are the merging of spirit and matter that may have nothing to do with the speed of breathing nor the size of your breath. The state of spiritual enlightenment and intuitive guidance of your breathing teacher or yourself is the biggest factor in determining the power of the energy flows. You have to experiment to know the truth about this. The energy flows are often subjectively described as a tingling or vibrating sensation throughout part or the whole body.

The energy flows are the process of filling your body with pure life energy and cleaning your mind and body of tension and impurities. Conscious breathing has the potential of cleaning the physical body and emotional body and nourishing them more efficiently than food.

Conscious breathing can give you a physical experience of spirit; a physiological experience of the human aura.

Conscious breathing is not a brand name, it is breathing consciously. It is a potential ability that you have always had. You can activate this ability by meditating on your breathing rhythm. It is probably the unconscious fear of psycho-physical memories that keeps people from discovering this power more frequently. Without understanding the hyperventilation symptoms that breath meditation can activate, it is easy to be frightened by your own mind. Of course, you will have to live out the drama of your psycho-physical memories anyway. But people have traditionally preferred the slow, fearful, painful way. Conscious breathing is fast, efficient, almost totally pleasurable, and amazing. When you are breathing right, it is not an effort, nor difficult. Right breathing is always natural and pleasurable. Conscious breathing is an inspiration, not a discipline. There is a wonderful power from within that supplies a special energy to maintain the breathing rhythm. This special energy is the Breath of Life, it is a healing and nourishing energy and it is always available to you, by meditating on the source of your breath as you keep your inhale connected to your exhale in an unbroken circle. The unity of the breath induces a physical experience of the unity of Being.

You can only learn the secrets of breathing from the Breath of Life itself—while breathing.

The Energy Body

Conscious maintenance of your energy body can keep you in a perpetual state of health and bliss and high personal energy. Most people are ignorant of the fact they they even have an energy body, much less how to take care of it. The basic purpose of conscious breathing is to clean and balance your energy body on a daily basis. This is as important as bathing, brushing your teeth or eating food. Everybody does connected breathing in the middle of deep sleep; it's what makes sleep work. The benefits of doing connected breathing while fully awake and conscious are greater than the benefits of sleep. Bathing helps to clean the energy body, sleep helps to balance it, and the right amount of food maintains energy. More people kill themselves from overeating than from starvation every year. Fasting is a valuable art to master for mental and physical health. In other words, the right amount of food is usually less. I recommend fasting one day per week for beginners for at least a year. It is safe and beneficial to limit fasting to one day per week (juices are OK) until you are well acquainted with your own body rhythms.

Benefits of Conscious Breathing

The daily practice of conscious breathing maintains a profound sense of spiritual and physical well-being. The conscious breathing ability gives you a great self-healing power that has healed everything known and unknown. It raises self-esteem and personal intelligence. It has also healed most "incurable diseases." Breathing is the great healer; stop breathing and you will get very, very sick.

Conscious breathing gives you a quick recovery ability that can be used during and between flights. It reduces absenteeism in airlines and other companies, especially after a person has completed ten sessions and can be called a conscious breather. It also helps employees fulfill their promises of friendliness and service. The conscious breathing rhythm can bring about the immediate cessation from pain and the ability to help spontaneously hyperventilating passengers.

A completed conscious breathing energy cycle cleans the nervous system and the circulatory system as well as the energy body. It may take only a few minutes or only a few hours to feel clean and balanced each time it is practiced.

The First Ten Sessions

If you have not been practicing the conscious, connected breathing rhythm on a daily basis like eating, then you can save yourself tons of discomfort, and perhaps prevent much pain, misery, and illness by doing at least ten one-hour to two-hour sessions with a well-trained breathing teacher or guide.

A session is usually done in a reclining position so that the body is relaxed. The purpose of each session is to guide the breathing rhythm until a completed energy cycle is achieved. The first five to twenty completed energy cycles, done perhaps one per week, seem to clear out enough physical tension and emotional blocks to enable people to practice conscious breathing alone. But having a breathing guide for the first ten sessions is of great value.

Teachers charge from $1 to $150 per session, depending upon their self-esteem and your ability to pay—it's negotiable. Investing the equivalent of a month's rent for ten simple breathing lessons is probably the best investment you will ever make. You can use the benefits forever. If you try to do it yourself and get stuck or afraid, it is obviously best to get a teacher. But if you have discomfort, you can try the breathing rhythm after a night's sleep—a little each day until you feel safe with it and can feel the results. To be afraid of your own breath leads to death. It is not possible to get the same benefits yourself that you can receive from the presence and guidance of a good breathing teacher.

Twenty Connected Breaths

Try twenty connected breaths, pulling softly on the inhale and relaxing on the exhale. Count them in groups of five, and on the fifth one fill all the room you can find in your body with your inhale. Breathe into your chest, your belly, your head, and your toes, but release the exhale immediately when full without any holding. Doing twenty connected breaths once or twice a day is totally safe.

Practical Goals

Each airline company can have its own breathing teachers. Many airline personnel have already been trained in conscious breathing, but require support from headquarters. Conscious breathing should be included in standard training programs for airline personnel. As it becomes more popular, it will be shared by individuals on a friendship basis, which has already started.

Conscious breathing should also be taught in our educational system at all levels. It should be taught in industry. The quality of life and work everywhere will improve dramatically when people learn how to breathe.

Physical Immortality

Any intelligent philosophy or perspective on life must deal with the fear of death and the prospect of physical immortality. Since breathing makes people more intelligent and enriches our personal aliveness, it is necessary to look at this question.

The idea of physical immortality can add another dimension to airline safety, and beyond safety to pleasure. To take the idea of physical immortality seriously as an actual possibility is outrageous. To start with, I'd like to say that it should not be taken seriously, but humorously. However, with 747s and space travel, why not?

The belief that death is inevitable has killed more people than all other causes combined. There are case histories of people living for thousands of years by practicing simple arts of spiritual purification, but you would never think of looking for them, if you didn't believe in physical immortality.

1. The philosophy of physical immortality. The belief that death is inevitable will kill you if nothing else does. But the truth is that your spirit is already eternal, you only have to move your mind and body into harmony with your eternal spirit.

2. The psychology of physical immortality. Unless your parents are already immortal, you have probably inherited a death urge. This personal death urge will kill you if you don't kill it. You kill it by unravelling your negative thoughts and feelings about life one at a time. Death has no power except what you give it in your own mind. Nobody can kill you but you. No one can kill you without your consent. Life is stronger than death. Your love is stronger than evil.

3. The physiology of physical immortality. It is obviously necessary to have a practical mastery of the physical body. In the West, a wonderful series of body techniques was evolved to make body mastery easy. Breath mastery, mastery of food, sleep, and physical pleasure are basic common denominators. But the truth is, it is easier than you think, "People have made spiritual mastery

so difficult, even God couldn't make it." But God has constructed man and woman so that eternal life is simple and natural. In the East, Yogic sciences have many ways of mastering the human body. The things that work the best are the most pleasurable. Spiritual purification is pleasurable because it is doing the things that are in harmony with our very nature.

The biggest cause of human body death is probably the denial or ignorance of your natural divinity and thus the misuse of the power of the human mind through negative thinking. The second biggest cause of death is probably inhibited breathing, which causes deprivation of oxygen to the blood, arteries, heart, brain, other organs and cells. The third biggest cause of body death is probably overeating, which pollutes the bloodstream. Three meals per day is the secret to death, not health. Moderate fasting not only improves health and aliveness, but also seems to reverse the aging process. The predominant scientific theory of agiing is excess cell pollution, which seems to be caused by overeating and under breathing. Filling the body with plenty of oxygen and spiritual energy through conscious breathing cleans the cells.

You are already immortal, until you prove otherwise: *Dying is more difficult than living.* The following affirmation has saved thousands of people from death. I recommend that you memorize it and master it through meditation. Mastering this affirmation now is like having your own personal guardian angel to protect you. Thoughts are angels.

"I am alive now, therefore my life urges are stronger than my death urges. As long as I strengthen my life urges and weaken my death urges, I will go on living in increasing health and youthfulness."

I unravelled my personal death urge in 1968. When I started teaching groups and training other professional group leaders and breathing coaches in 1974, I realized that I needed more than a weekend to permit the quality of personal transformation I was interested in stimulating. Therefore, I created a one-year seminar program, which is a simple form consisting of the same people meeting as a group for one whole day, usually from 10 a.m. to 10 p.m., once a month for one year. The basic purpose of the group is to provide a safe supportive environment for people to realize their natural divinity. To keep a group like this together for one year with a full discussion of the most intimate human issues has been more successful than marriages, statistically, because of the simple quality of the ideas they are based on.

Today these groups exist all over the world and produce high-quality human lives, people who enjoy themselves. In the real world, temporary insanity is a popular fad, as everyone can see. Temporary insanity has almost become socially acceptable! As a result of working with these groups for six years, I have written a book called *Physical Immortality, the Science of Everlasting Life,* which is published by Celestial Arts. This book expands all the ideas included in this booklet. It includes pictures of an actual immortal who has mastered his body for over 600 years.

Flight crews and other company groups who work together for a year are, in fact, a one-year seminar. This book can increase the quality of their communication, relationships, productivity and happiness.

Spiritual enlightenment enables people to take charge of their lives. The ideas of spiritual enlightenment are very simple and are widely available today in books, tapes, magazines and seminars.

The ideas that produce spiritual enlightenment can be expressed in many different ways. Here are two very brief ways.

1. Thought is creative and you are the thinker. The ability to think is universal. There is one thinker in the universe and you are a thinking center in this one thinker. The physical universe and your personal reality are created by your thoughts, conscious or unconscious. When you realize this and raise the quality of your thoughts enough to produce a world that you personally enjoy, you can call yourself spiritually enlightened. All human misery, sickness, violence, and death are caused by ignorance of the Law of Mind. The Law of Mind is that thought is creative whether we believe it or not. To live without being consciously responsible for the quality of our thoughts is to misuse the power of the human mind.

2. Infinite Being, Infinite Intelligence, and Infinite Manifestation. Infinite Being is the space between your thoughts—spirit, life itself, the Source, God, Shiva, Allah, Christ. Your next thought can go anywhere in the whole of Infinite Knowledge. Your mind is always centered in either Infinite Intelligence or Infinite Stupidity, whether you realize it or not. You have approximately 50,000 creative thoughts every day that maintain your feelings and circumstances. You can change them if you don't like what you see. Infinite Manifestation is your body, your personal reality including your emotions, and the big, beautiful world out there. The physical universe exists for the purpose of supporting your spirit, mind and body in comfort and pleasure forever.

Your mind has a personal law at all times. A personal law is one thought that dominates your mind and life more than any other thought. The Five Biggies are common denominators of personal laws: (1) birth trauma; (2) parental disapproval syndrome; (3) specific negatives; (4) unconscious death urge; (5) past lives. Examining your life in light of the Five Biggies can increase understanding and self-improvement very rapidly.

Affirmations and Goals

The human mind is usually being misused when it is not used consciously and purposefully. Goals and affirmations can easily enable you to use your mind consciously to create a beautiful reality for yourself and others around you at all times. To be clear about your goals in life, make a list of at least one hundred things you would like to have, be or achieve (things, qualities, activities).

The affirmation principle involves choosing your own thoughts and using them with enough repetition to make their creative power work in the real world. An example of a good affirmation is "I am highly pleasing to myself in the presence of other people." When I was working as a consciousness consultant counselling individuals, I sold this affirmation for $50 per person and when the people who bought it wrote the affirmation on paper 20 times a day for one month, they got their money's worth.

The Death Urge and Physical Immortality

An airline flight magazine reported a few years ago that 50 percent of commercial pilots die within two years after retirement. Why? I have a few theories. The many thousands of people who have completed a one-year seminar have exposed the death urge and how it works. Your personal death urge can be viewed as a psychic entity that will kill you if you don't kill it first. If your parents are not physically immortal, you probably inherited a death urge. You can unravel your death urge one thought at a time by changing deathist mentality to aliveness mentality. You start by questioning the long-held and popular belief that death is inevitable and beyond your control. Obviously, pilots as a profession have not yet ascended into the upper regions of spiritual enlightenment. On the other hand, the unconscious self-improvement stimulus of regular flying is pushing their minds to do so. The tension of deathist mentality is suppressed in the interest of keeping the job and maintaining the safety of their passengers and planes, which of course are worthy purposes.

Pilots have a reputation of being straight, conventional, uptight, sane, upper-middle-class, intelligent and dependable. Pilots have traditionally held themselves together by force of mind until they retire. Then they relax and are overwhelmed by so much personal negativity that they die in two years.

Temporary insanity prevents permanent death! Obviously, pilots need to create within their profession procedures for safely and successfully handling temporary insanity and the death urge without endangering their careers and their passengers. A first step is to permit absence from work for emotional illness to be as socially acceptable as it is for physical illness. I believe that all physical illness is caused by neglected emotional illness. This means that people who are physically ill are chronically emotionally ill. It also means that consciously dealing with emotional disturbances make people permanently healthy.

Realistically, each person needs a "spiritual enlightenment adjustment period" at some time in their life during which time personal divinity becomes a practical responsibility. It is the time in history for humans to evolve from animal to divine. We can no longer stifle personal divinity in the interest of corporate profits. Airlines and other companies must teach spiritual enlightenment and enough self-improvement principles to enable their employees to become self-realized beings. Employees, including the ones who are already supposed to have it together, must be given the space for temporary insanity. Otherwise, the result is permanent death.

The amazing thing is that when people let a few of these simple, if radical, concepts and practices into their minds and lives, everything works better. People who think through the ideas of physical immortality report quantum jumps in health, success, love, satisfaction, productivity, energy and aliveness. It feels good to stop killing yourself and everyone around you with your negative thoughts. But to keep yourself in mortal mindedness is to perpetuate gloom and doom.

Conscious thinking, conscious breathing, a little body work, spiritual purification, loving service to others, and spiritual community are the "non-secrets" to happy and successful human existence.

Obviously, airline personnel must be happy humans first, before airplanes can be happy places. In all labor surveys I have ever read, self-determination, good relationships, freedom of thought and speech, and the intangible spiritual context of the work environment were always valued more highly by employees than money. I fly so much that I have a vested interest in upgrading the "vibes" in airplanes. I hope these ideas get widely distributed, discussed and implemented.

Achieving physical immortality takes more than a superficial mouthing of the philosophy. I'd suggest that you seek out and study with some actual immortal. Without the idea you'd never look for the. In September 1980 I found out about two immortals in India. In 57 B.C., Babaji gave physical immortality to two persons. Bhartreeji, one of them, was a king at the time. Since then, he has lived in a forest a few hours drive west of Delhi. He has come out into the public at least once every hundred years to teach the people by doing miracles. We are really proud of our comfortable and affluent Western lifestyle, but India has thousands of lifestyles that we haven't even thought of yet.

Babaji is the eternal manifestation of spirit in human form who has maintained a residence in the Himalayas near Halwani since the world started. Guidance to his ashram can be received from the Kalash View Hotel in Haldwani. He has always been available to us throughout human history on earth. But people have habitually been more interested in ignorance and death than in the yogic sciences of mind and body mastery. Today, however, comfort, pleasure, education, affluence, mechanical technology, and universal government have expanded the mind of the average person to the point that killing ourselves is more difficult to keep a secret. We have unconsciously created the context for self-mastery. The alternatives are nuclear war, or snipers on middle-class suburban streets. Perhaps truth, simplicity, and love are more inevitable than death.

I have been saddened over the years by spiritually enlightened groups that don't teach physical immortality. To raise your consciousness means to free yourself from negative thoughts, but if you never question mortal mentality, then the statistical results reveal that your fear of death will haunt you until you kill yourself. On the other hand, if you believe that life beyond the grave is better than the here and now, you have double motivation for death. A moment's thought would reveal that the here and now is the same without a body as in one, and that the value of physical death is highly over-rated.

The pilot's retirement and death statistics indicate that flying unconsciously evolves pilots spiritually and, without conscious knowledge of the death urge, they become victimized by it very rapidly. A very plausible theory to explain plane accidents is that a passenger load dominated by deathist mentality can cause mechanical failure just as the mind can cause a body organ failure or natural disasters. The human mind is the same mind in essence as the mind of God and is therefore infinitely powerful! This is true whether we acknowledge it or not.

It is also possible that pilots and other members of the flight crew process the deathist mentality of passengers, as well as other forms of negativity. This is done telephatically in the course of a normal work day. Airline personnel are therapists, consciously or unconsciously, for everyone on the plane. It is amazing to me that they survive so well. They are advanced beings.

I have been thinking about these things over the years and have felt frustrated by the lack of communication between myself and the airline personnel that I trust my body to and pay well to keep safe while I experience the pleasure and convenience of speedy exalted travel. I'm willing to teach in-training departments, and to counsel executives, pilots, and flight attendants on all levels, including sales, maintenance and construction. Obviously, I can't personally do all the teaching that needs to be done, but I have trained a few thousand capable teachers who are available to serve airlines around the world.

A few ideas for spreading this information: I have no fear about telling the truth to people because I have noticed that their natural divinity can handle it.

1. Put this book into plane seat pockets and see if it gets "stolen" more frequently than flight magazines. I bet it becomes more popular than peanuts.

2. Through my publisher, I will give my permission to have it published in flight magazines for standard author fees. I'm willing to read or have it read as a stereo program.

3. Provide seminars for working personnel.

4. "Start temporary insanity programs while in training school." I am attempting to state this humorously. Actually temporary insanity started with airline personnel in childhood. The tragic paradox is that businesses pretend that emotional illness

doesn't exist, and this pretense multiplies the tension to the breaking point. People can only stuff their feelings so long, then they quit. The positive side of this paradox is that profits, job satisfaction, efficiency and dependability increase when businesses acknowledge the natural divinity of their people as well as their emotional problems. It doesn't pay to lie about our human emotions, positive or negative, in the name of profit and social acceptability.

5. It is time for a "spiritual liberation" movement in business.

6. Airlines must become more conscious about sales expansion from the standpoint of air pollution. Quality of personnel and service might be more important than sales expansion. I've noticed that sales expansion naturally comes out of quality and declines rapidly when quality is missing. Airlines have a vested interest in solving automobile air pollution problems to make room for their own.

7. The airlines have perhaps unconsciously done more to promote world peace than the United Nations. Air travel builds global consciousness and breaks up blind nationalism. I'd like to see a universal international exchange program at the high-school level. Airlines have a vested interest in promoting this.

The people I have trained to teach freedom of thought, conscious breathing, etc., are available throughout the world. Some are self-trained, others are just aware and are experimenting. It is up to you to teach yourself and to be responsible for the quality of the teachers that you choose. I recommend that you don't limit yourself to one teacher and that you have an in-depth and complete relationship with your spiritual teachers that is as rich or richer than blood family. The realization of the one spiritual family can create heaven on earth. It's worth thinking about.

Water Purification

I finished the last few pages of this while lying in my bathtub. My favorite self-improvement technique is thinking and breathing in a warm bathtub. It amazes me how many freedoms are guaranteed in the U.S. Constitution (as well as the U.S.S.R. Constitution) that people don't use. Our abundance of hot water doesn't nourish us if we don't use it. Our freedom of speech doesn't free us if we don't use it, and our New Age technology doesn't free us if we don't use it. Likewise, our natural divinity doesn't make us happy, healthy, and wealthy as long as we try to separate it from business.

Breathing is air purification, fasting is earth purification, meditating on a candle or fireplace is fire purification, and bathing is water purification. Earth, air, water and fire are the basic physical elements of the human body and the universe. Here are a few suggestions for conscious bathing.

After a flight, or anytime I am with a group of people in any situation, I always run for my bathtub as soon as possible. I always say to the people who greet me, "Take me to your bathtub." The purpose of daily bathing is more to clean my energy body than my skin. If you breathe and think slowly, and enter the water slowly, you will become aware of your invisible energy body (or emotional body).

In other words, fill your tub, step into it, relax, think and breathe before sitting down in the water. You will notice physical and emotional feelings change in your consciousness. Next, sit down slowly into the water without losing awareness of your breath and feelings. Breathe for a few minutes in the sitting position in a relaxed way. Then lay back with the water up to your neck and covering your chest, without losing consciousness of your breathing and feelings. To complete, put the top of your head and your forehead under the water, with you nose and mouth out, still breathing and being aware of your feelings—both physical and emotional.

You may notice spots or bands of energy concentrate in your body and then change, transform, or dissolve as you continue to think and breathe. This is the normal sensation that occurs when you clean and balance your energy body with water and breath. I find it fun and interesting to observe the psychic dirt and tensions and negative feelings disappear as I practice this simple method of spiritual purification. I usually do it twice a day, before and after sleeping. Babaji once told me that sleep is death and that bathing after sleep washes the death off my soul. I usually take from fifteen minutes to perhaps several hours of relaxing in the water until I feel good and the energy centers of my body feel clean and balanced.

If you have unusual experiences that you don't understand, please feel free to write me with your comments and questions.

I've found that my personal income is higher than pilots and most business executives as a result of constantly telling the truth about my personal divinity as well as my most negative thoughts and feelings. In other words, personal spiritual purification does not inhibit business success, it is the secret to getting rich!

If you desire to know whether or not I am immortal or if anyone else is, there is only one way to know for sure. You will have to stick around and see.

Renewal of the Money System

I've tried to write about this before. It is the idea on which Prosperity International was based. As far as I know it has never been expressed before in print. I keep working at simpler and clearer ways of expressing it. This is another attempt.

We are the source of the money system. Money is printed by us. In order for the money system to work we have to distribute to every person in the economy a supply of money. To keep the money system working we have to distribute a supply of money to every person in the economy regularly. The money system must experience renewal. We must resurrect our responsibility for the money system which we have delegated to the Federal government and use it more rationally.

We have permitted our money system to be used without much intelligent control from us, the authors of it. We must realize that money is our servant, not our master. Money has traditionally been used by one person or group to gain power over others and mainly it is used today with short sighted ignorance.

Money is a means of exchange. Money is not wealth, it is a means of exchanging wealth. Wealth is the ideas, goods and services that we produce. Without wealth money would be useless because there would be nothing to buy. Obviously the regular distribution of money to everyone should be related to the total value of the goods and services we are producing. We, the producers, the distributors, and the consumers of wealth are the source of money. We invented and use money for the purpose of facilitating the exchange of the ideas, goods and services that we create. Money works, it is a wonderful invention, but it only works properly when we, the creators of it, the printers of it, give ourselves a regular supply so we can stay in the money game.

This principle was practiced in some cultures who evolved their money system in a more conscious way. The U.S. money system was not evolved rationally by a person or group who understood what money was. I have looked in ancient as well as modern literature about money and never found an adequate discussion of what money is and how a money system is supposed to work. So I decided to meditate on it until I separated the myth from the reality so I could put justice into money—common sense.

The purpose of producing ideas, goods and services is not to earn money. The purpose in nature of producing ideas, goods and services is to have the ideas, goods and services to consume or enjoy. When we produce more ideas, goods and services than we can use ourselves we share them with other people. However, some people produce ideas, goods and services not for the purpose of consuming them themselves, but rather because they have the ability to produce them. In other words, a complex economy with a money system permits specialization to the point where people no longer have to produce for their own needs. They can produce for many reasons. People produce for artistic reasons. They produce for the purpose of accumulating larger bank balances. People produce sometimes for survival but the self-sufficient person who lives directly off the land is rare. In fact, to be self-sufficient means to farm your own food, to make your own clothes and shelter without using any tools produced by other people. Do you have the ability to make your own matches?

PART III

More Ideas for a New Age

Practical Applications of Creative Thought and Rebirthing in Special Areas of Your Life

8 Money in Abundance

All human wealth is created by the human mind, and being wealthy is a function of enlightenment. Forget about hard work and struggling to get ahead—the way to increase your income is by increasing the quality of your ideas. The most important attribute you can bring to the creation of your own personal wealth is a well-developed prosperity consciousness, which is a structure of positive ideas about money. This, in turn, is based in your positive self-esteem. With these qualities you will carry your prosperity around with you and create it wherever you go.

Your mind is a machine, and it will produce wealth as easily as poverty. One of the basic laws of the mind is the "law of increase"; whatever you concentrate on increases. If you concentrate on the fun you are having with your money, then your money will increase and your fun will too. If you concentrate on the misery your money gives you, then your misery will increase.

It is important to collect good ideas, either from seminars, books or your own personal connection to Infinite Intelligence, then work with those ideas through affirmations. A suggested affirmation is, "I deserve to be prosperous and wealthy." You must have enough self-esteem to believe that you deserve it; then, no matter how much you have, you will enjoy it. Many wealthy people are unhappy because they unconsciously feel they don't deserve their prosperity and success. Probably the most powerful affirmation you can work with to double your income is a self-esteem affirmation that says, "I am highly pleasing to myself in the presence of other people."

Money always follows your instructions! If you don't like the way money is behaving for you, then change your instructions. This chapter will suggest some new instructions that will work for you if you instill them as causative factors in your consciousness.

To build a prosperity consciousness, it is important for you to know the four laws of wealth:

1. The Earning Law (or production law)
2. The Spending Law (or giving law)
3. The Savings Law
4. The Investing Law

If you master all four of these laws, then becoming a millionaire is inevitable.

The Earning Law

You will never make big money working just for money.

It is a paradox that only when you give up money as a motivation will you start making big money. What works is to find out what you really enjoy doing in life, the thing you have always loved doing, the thing you have always wanted to do with your time, and then figure out how to make money doing it. When you enjoy what you are doing, people will enjoy paying you money for it. If you don't enjoy what you are doing, then what good is money, anyway? If you dedicate yourself to making money in the hope of saving enough to have a good time in the future, the future never seems to come.

In Leonard's case, he enjoyed sitting home reading deeply profound metaphysical books, and he started to spend more time doing just that. For one month he sat home and read, while working in sales only about half as much as before. At the end of the month he had tripled his income. When you realized he had done this by working half as much, he became clear that what counts isn't how much time you put in, but rather the quality of your thoughts and ideas. What happened was that he raised his self-esteem. He realized that his customers wanted to know about the subjects he was studying. Some were so interested that they offered to pay him, saying they did not have time to read. The first to offer to pay him was a lawyer making $50,000 a year. He paid Leonard twenty dollars an hour to share what he had been reading. Then Leonard got the idea of guaranteeing his friends, to whom he had been "giving" his knowledge anyway, a 50 percent increase in income within twelve weeks if they took a four-week course from him for which he would charge eighty dollars. One friend was making fifteen hundred dollars a month. At the end of the first month, he made thirty-three hundred dollars and at the end of the second month, forty-five hundred dollars. He was very happy with the results. When Leonard saw that his friends were paying him eighty dollars per month and making thousands of dollars, he figured he was selling himself too cheaply and increased the rates to fifty dollars per hour. (When you become self-employed you have the right to set your own value on your services.) Not so surprisingly, at this point Leonard found that people were even more willing to pay fifty dollars an hour than he was willing to receive it.

In our economy you can make money doing anything. Make a list of the things you enjoy doing most in life. This will stimulate your imagination, and you make money with your imagination. The people who are really working for money in our economy are the people who spend forty hours a week for forty years and end up broke at age sixty-five, living on Social Security. The people who are having the most fun winning the money game are those who aren't working for money. The ones who are working for money "bad-mouth" the people who aren't working for money because they have more money. Beautiful paradox, right?

After you make enough money to become financially independent and you don't have to work for money, why work then? The people who don't have money assume that those other people would go to the beach. The fact is, they *did* go to the beach until that became more work than working. They sat around for awhile and then they came to the realization that the thing they really liked to do was what they were doing, and so they make money in spite of themselves.

We repeat, the easiest way to make money is to do the thing you enjoy doing. Make a list of your ten greatest pleasures and figure out how to make money at a couple of them. No matter what it is that you think of that you enjoy doing, you can think of someone who has or is making money doing that.

Money is nothing but pieces of paper with symbols and numbers; and, originally, money was nothing more than an idea in a person's mind. Actually, you can get everything you want without money. The perfect example of that is a woman who calls herself "Peace Pilgrim." She has been walking across the country for more than twenty years, having vowed to walk until there is peace throughout the world. She never, ever begs for money. She has developed a prosperity consciousness (that ultimate trust in the universe that the universe will support you) and today she can go to cities anywhere and take her pick of any number of mansions to stay in. She is not only chauffeured around, but also constantly has to turn down money. Sometimes people give her material things which she has to turn away. So you can sell all your possessions and live without money altogether.

The other end of the spectrum is to seek money directly. Leonard has an idea that will be worth one million dollars in cash to you at the end of the year. What you have to do is interview a multi-millionaire once a day. What you do is to offer the millionaire an idea that is worth a million dollars. There are approximately 500,000 millionaires in the country so you have lots of opportunities. All you have to do is meet with four a week for fifty weeks. Multimillionaires would love to spend a million on an idea that is valuable enough. When you spend time with people who already have a prosperity consciousness, it will rub off on you. Most people have difficulty thinking of an idea worth a million dollars. If you do have difficulty, on your first interview ask the first millionaire to give you ten ideas that would be worth a million dollars to him. All you have to do is qualify for one of the ten. It is just a question as to whether you have enough self-esteem to call up a millionaire and ask him that stupid question.

It is important to understand that the more wealth is created, the more wealth there is to go around. The more millionaires there are, the easier it is to become a millionaire. So don't resent millionaires.

The affirmations for the *earning law* are:

1. I deserve to be prosperous and wealthy.
2. My job is the pipeline by which I tap the infinite wealth of my United States economy for my own personal use.
3. My personal connection to Infinite Being and Infinite Intelligence is adequate enough to yield a huge personal fortune.

The last affirmation is one of the most valuable ideas in the universe. If you are connected to Infinite Intelligence, then you have access to all other ideas in the universe. That, in essence, is what Leonard learned from all those metaphysical books.

The Spending Law

The purpose of money is to spend it and money has a way of multiplying when you spend it. The spending law is all about the art of negotiating. There are three affirmations for the spending law:

1. Every dollar I spend comes back to me multiplied.
2. My income now exceeds my expenses.
3. The more willing I am to prosper other people, the more willing other people are to prosper me.

Consider the first affirmation. If you take a dollar and spend it with Richard, then you give a dollar for Richard's merchandise and he gets your dollar. He takes your dollar and spends it with John. John spends it with Carol and it goes on through ten transactions, until the tenth person who gets your dollar spends it with you. So you get your dollar back, plus a dollar's worth of

Richard's merchandise. Everybody is one dollar richer because they each earned and spent your dollar, thereby gaining one dollar's worth of whatever they desired. Superficially it looks as if you didn't create wealth, but just moved it, acquiring the material thing or service that was important to you. But you did *produce* something to sell to the tenth person. Consumption and an ongoing exchange process increase production. Spending money is actually a productive function.

Leonard's definition of profit is "the creation of new wealth by the arbitrary decree of the individual business person." So let's look at some other transactions. Richard sells books for one dollar that he buys for fifty cents. The moment you gave him one dollar, his book had doubled in value. If each of the ten people had a piece of merchandise worth fifty cents and sold it for a dollar, then through the transaction they turned five dollars worth of merchandise into ten dollars worth of wealth. They arbitrarily created five dollars worth of new wealth out of nothing. So, every time you circulate your money, more personal wealth is created. *All spending is giving.*

To become a millionaire yourself, working on a 10 percent profit margin, you will have to create nine million dollars for other people. That means that every person who is becoming a millionaire is creating money for you. If your objective is to become a millionaire and everybody you do business with is only making $5,000 per year, you will have to do business with a lot of people in order to make a million. But if you had 500,000 millionaires to do business with, you don't have to do business with very many to make a million. The more millionaires there are, the easier it is for you to make a million. When you have a million, the only thing to do with it is to spend it. Our economy multiplies it even faster because if you put your money in a bank or savings and loan company, they will spend that money at least once while you are collecting interest on it. They loan it out to a person with a worthy project and the person they loan it to spends it.

The value of money is determined by the buyer and seller in every transaction, so the value of money is renegotiated during every transaction. Millionaires not only value money, but they are also the best negotiators; this is because they are not financially embarrassed. Poor people as a rule don't negotiate because they don't have enough self-esteem, in addition to which they are embarrassed about money. The value of everything is ultimately intuitive.

The second affirmation, "My income now exceeds my expenses," is true for you because right now you have an excess of money. If you have any money in your pocket, purse, bank or anywhere, then you have an excess of money. But how often do you give yourself credit for having this excess? Probably you go around saying that your bills exceed your income—and they don't! The proof is in your pocket. In every person's consciousness there is a surplus somewhere in their own personal wealth. Right now you have a surplus of money. If you concentrate on this surplus it will spread throughout all your financial affairs. (On the other hand, if you concentrate on the lack, lack can spread—but not quite as easily. It is harder to spread lack than surplus because surplus is in harmony with nature. If surplus was not in harmony with nature, there wouldn't be a universe!) So, what have YOU been concentrating on? The bills? Have they gotten bigger? *The basic law of the mind is the law of increase.* So it obviously behooves you to develop a "surplus consciousness." If you concentrate on your surplus, your surplus will get bigger. Another way of expressing this metaphysical law is like this: *Whatever you think about expands.*

The way to master this concept is to play a little game called the "percentage monthly budget game " One purpose of this game is to demonstrate to yourself that you create money and you can solve your financial problems with imagination. Make a list of all the categories and things you want to spend money on: food, rent, entertainment, transportation, self-improvement, savings, bills, clothes, whatever. (Do NOT have a category for emergencies. You don't want to "set yourself up" for emergencies.) Next, establish a percentage of your income to be budgeted for each category. Look at how you spent your money for the past month. Suppose you're making $1000 per month and you spend 20 percent on food, 20 percent on rent, etc. At the beginning of the month, arbitrarily change at least two of these category percentages. Look at the categories and pick out which ones you want to try changing. Let's say you want to stay in the same apartment that you are in. You can increase your rent to 25 percent and produce a surplus of fifty dollars, but you have to reduce something else. Let's say you decide to cut your food budget in half and spend only 10 percent on food. That gives you an extra 10 percent, which you can put in one of the other categories, or you can divide it among them so you have a surplus in every category. The prize for winning the game and producing a surplus is that you can take all the surpluses and blow them!

Now that leaves you with a problem for your imagination, which is to eat better on half as much money. There are hundreds of solutions. One is to call up seven of your friends and ask them how they would like to have you for dinner once a week. If you have enough self-esteem, that won't be a problem. Or have ten of your friends come to your house for dinner and charge them less than if they went to a restaurant.

Let's take a look at the priorities on which people spend their money. What comes first? The rent: and this is the worst investment on the list. Compare rent with self-improvement. You paid $5.95 for this book and you get to use this information forever. The fact is that self-improvement is the most valuable item of your budget and most people don't even have a category for it. Fear of running out causes you to spend only on things people told you to spend money on. When it comes to buying things that are really good for you and that make you happy, guilt comes. When you say, "I don't have enough money to go to that self-improvement seminar, or buy that self-improvement book" it is almost like saying, "I am not a good investment." The best way to make money is to invest in yourself, and that is what self-improvement is all about. So take a look at re-doing your budget and making self-improvement the top priority. That is what I did. It works.

Another technique to increase your prosperity consciousness is to carry a big bill. Work up to a $100 bill. The rule is that you can't spend it unless you can replace it instantly. That means you always have to have $100 in your possession all the time—and you start thinking "rich." Everytime you look in your billfold, you have that hundred, and you get used to always having plenty of money. When you are able to replace it, spend it just for fun and then go get another one to teach your mind that there is no sense of loss. It puts you in a position of strength if you have a large bill and you don't have to spend it. Before I tried this, back when I was afraid I'd lose big bills, I would open my billfold and have a thought like this: "I am running out." Since thoughts are creative, I was programming myself for poverty. Now when I open my billfold and see the $100 bill in there, I think: "Oh, I still have a hundred. I have plenty." Or, "I have enough money." Furthermore, when you give up your theft consciousness and your fear of loss, nobody ever steals from you and you never lose your billfold or purse!

It is important to remember that all spending is giving; and it is a good idea to say to yourself when you open a bill that has to be paid, *"Oh good, a chance to outflow!"* If you see spending or paying bills as a loss, you are headed for trouble. "Give and it shall be given unto you." Get into the spirit of spending. Also, remember that bills are agreements. Try negotiating them if you have lots of old bills, at least until you develop a surplus consciousness.

Most people think that their budget is a function of their income. If you win at the budget game for three to six consecutive months, then your income will become a function of your budget. This means that you can raise your budget a realistic amount and your income will go up to match it automatically. If you arbitrarily increase your budget by 10 percent, your mind will begin to create the money—on the street or anywhere, mystically and magically. Once your mind accepts the fact that your income always exceeds your expenses, when you raise your expenses your mind will create the money to match.

The Savings Law

There are two affirmations for the Savings Law:
1. A part of all I earn is mine to keep (save).

2. Every day my income increases whether I am working, playing or sleeping.

If you have money in a savings account, then your money is increasing every day whether you are working, playing or sleeping, so the affirmations are already true. Once your mind has accepted the savings law on this basic level, it will transfer it to all other levels. The way you practice the Savings Law is to have at least four savings accounts:

1. Large Purchases
2. Investment
3. Annual Income
4. Financial Independence

(1) *Large purchases.* The basic goal is to keep this account empty, and it is extremely difficult to do that when you have the other three savings accounts. When you have a real prosperity consciousness, you will create the money you intended to draw out of the savings account before you have time to get to the bank.

(2) *Investment capital.* Everyone at one point has thought of owning stock or real estate; and most people don't have any. The reason most people don't have any is because they don't have an investment savings account. You have probably never had enough money together at one time to invest in the stock market or to buy real estate. So that is the purpose of this account; and you cannot withdraw money from it for anything but investments that pay a higher rate of return. The savings account must be governed by this rule.

(3) *Annual income.* There are two purposes for this account. The first is to accumulate an annual income so that you will have a year's income in reserve, and you can take a year off any time that you desire without working. The second purpose is to use the annual income account as your basic cash flow. In other words, you put all of your income into your annual income account, and then draw some out (less than you put in) for ongoing expenses. You make a weekly transfer from your savings account to your check-

ing account. This gives you a new kind of mentality because you learn that you have the ability to pay yourself.

Leonard invented this idea for a man who was making $70,000 per year. One day this man couldn't pay his bills, and when Leonard asked him how much his monthly expenses were, he did not know. Leonard told him that what he needed was an annual income account with at least $30,000 in it so he did not have to worry about working for a year. The man borrowed $30,000 and put it in that income account. He made $150,000 in six months after that, or doubled his income in half the time. What happened was that he didn't have to worry about money for a year, so that meant whenever he went on his regular "psychological problem cycle," it was not tied in with money. Always before, his psychological problems got tied up with his financial problems; he had though his psychological problems were financial problems. When he didn't have to worry about money for a year, he recognized his psychological problems for what they were; and so he solved them and doubled his income in less than half the time. If you do this, you can't get depressed about money, so you have to think about something else.

(4) *Financial Independence.* This is the most important savings account. The purpose of it is to accumulate enough income so you can live off the interest, whether you work or not. In order to make this account work, you need to abide by two rules: (a) You can *never* take out the principal. The money you deposit in that account has to stay there *forever.* (b) You have to spend a portion of the interest regularly.

If you are adding to the principal regularly, then you can take all the interest and spend it. If you stop adding to the principal, then you can only spend up to 90 percent of the interest. In this way, the interest check will get bigger and bigger all the time. Just having the reality of an interest check in your consciousness will blow your mind. Basic to this account is the necessity to figure out what financial independence means to you. What it means to Leonard is $1000 per month coming in whether he works or not.

You can have all savings accounts in one bank if it is more convenient for you. Every time you get a pay check, you can deposit it in the appropriate account(s). Every time you go to the bank, make a deposit. You should make a deposit in each one every month. It stimulates your imagination.

I heard this idea of the four savings accounts from Leonard when I first met him. I thought it sounded great and yet it took me a whole year to open them. Then it took me even longer to learn to use them regularly. I just wasn't used to saving. What I found worked best was to *pay myself first*, taking out money from my income for my savings accounts before anything else. I also found it useful to make a deposit in each account every single week. In this way I trained myself to develop good savings habits and become financially independent.

The Investment Law

There are two affirmations for this law:
1. All my investments are profitable.
2. Part of all my profits go into permanent wealth, current expenses, capital and reserves.

Your mind can just as easily make all your investments profitable as only half of them. Whatever you concentrate on increases, so if you concentrate on having only 50 percent of your investments profitable, then that is the way it will turn out. Divide your profits from each investment into four categories and place a portion in each:
1. Expenses
2. Investments
3. Investment savings account
4. Financial independence acccount

(1) *Expenses.* The purpose of spending a portion of each profit on each investment cycle is so that you build a consciousness of benefiting from your investment in the present instead of saving for the future (which never comes).

(2) *Investments.* If you take a portion of your profits and add it

to your original capital, then your original capital always gets bigger.

(3) *Investment savings account.* By putting a portion of your profit in this account, your investments always keep diversifying.

(4) *Financial independence savings account.* A part of your profits become permanent wealth in this account.

There is a lot more to say about these simple and powerful laws. Leonard's money tapes expand them a lot. Leonard may put out a whole book on the subject, but if you practice these laws for a year, you will be able to write a book yourself.

MONEY AFFIRMATIONS

Law 1—Earning Law

1. I deserve to be wealthy.
2. My job is the pipeline by which I tap the infinite wealth of my U.S. economy for my own personal desires.
3. My personal connection to Infinite Being and Infinite Intelligence is adequate enough to yield a huge personal fortune.

Law 2—Spending Law

1. My income now exceeds my expenses.
2. Every dollar I spend comes back to me multiplied.
3. The more willing I am to prosper others, the more willing others are to prosper me.
4. The more willing others are to prosper me, the more willing I am to prosper others.
5. I now have a positive personal cash flow.

Law 3—Savings Law

1. My income increases every day whether I am working, sleeping or playing.
2. A part of all I earn is mine to keep.

Law 4—Investing Law

1. All my investments are profitable.

2. Part of all my profits goes into permanent wealth, current expenses, capital and reserves.

MORE MONEY AFFIRMATIONS

1. I now have a success consciousness with money.
2. I now have a surplus consciousness.
3. I enjoy being economically self-sufficient.
4. People enjoy paying me money for what I enjoy doing the most.
5. Life always holds out as much goodness as I am willing to accept.
6. I am enjoying creating prosperity for the person who gives me money.
7. My connection to Infinite Intelligence is adequate enough to yield a huge personal fortune.
8. The more willing I am to prosper others, the more willing they are to prosper me.
9. I have the right to give myself permission to become wealthy or do anything I want.
10. I no longer have to go along with the erroneous ideas of my parents about making money.
11. The wealthier I become, the more I spread it around.
12. Each year my money increases faster than I spend it.
13. It takes less effort to be wealthy than it does to keep out the universal supply.
14. Life rewards me with abundance.
15. I deserve to be wealthy, rich, prosperous, affluent.
16. I enjoy expressing my abundance.
17. I now have a prosperity consciousness all of the time.
18. If I don't watch out, money will drop into my lap.
19. I don't have to work to get money.
20. Money is trying to come to me and, if I just get out of the way, it will happen.
21. People are now rewarding me with money just for being alive.

The Renewal of Money (by Leonard Orr)

Economics is based on production, distribution, and consumption. Money is a means of exchanging production. Money is not wealth, but a means of exchanging wealth. Wealth is ideas, goods and services.

Money is the grease of distribution. Money is a convenient substitute for direct barter. The purpose of money is to facilitate the consumption of our production. The purpose of money is to make it easier for consumers to use our production.

The basic principle which creates a money system in the nature of human economics is: Producers and consumers create money for the purpose of exchanging and using their ideas, goods, and services. The producers and consumers of ideas, goods and services are the source of money. We have the right to create a money system that works. We have the right to print and distribute money in a logical way.

To start a money system, money has to be printed and distributed among the producers and consumers on an equitable basis. The renewal of money can only happen when money is printed and distributed regularly. We, the producers and consumers of wealth, have authorized the Federal Govoernment to print money, but we did not authorize them to distribute money in a logical and equitable way on a regular basis that can allow the money system to work as it should. The people of most economies of the world, perhaps all, do not practice the basic principle of money intelligently. We are the source of money. We create the money system. It is our responsibility to build the principle of renewal into the money system by giving all participants in the economy a regular supply of money.

Every individual human should receive a regular supply of money so that the money system can continue to work for everyone. The purpose of production is consumption. If consumers do not have enough money to purchase the production, it is wasted. The producer as well as the consumer then loses the money game.

Money is not wealth. Production is wealth. Ideas, goods and services are production. Money is a means of exchanging production. In a money economy, if there is no production, money is worthless; and if there is no money, production is worthless. If consumers have no money, production is worthless. Production has no value until it is consumed. The health of the economy is production and consumption and money is the means of exchange between producers and consumers.

Money is printed by the Federal Government. For the money system to work logically and equitably, a regular monthly supply of money must be distributed to every person so each person can participate in the economy every month.

Money is worthless without production. Therefore, money should be distributed in proportion to production. Production is worthless without consumption. Therefore, for money to work, consumers must have a regular supply of money. Since consumers are people and every person is a consumer, every person deserves a regular supply of money. If consumers don't have money, production stops, in a money economy. If money is not redistributed regularly, consumption and production stops regularly.

Therefore, if we like to have a healthy economy, we have to get our government or our banks to distribute, to ourselves, a monthly supply of money.

In the past, money was given to consumers by producers and money was given to producers by consumers. It has always been assumed that this would work or, at least, that it *should* work. The truth is that sometimes it does work and sometimes it doesn't. It works when there is enough money in the hands of consumers and enough production in the hands of the producers. When people forget that they are the source and creators of both production and money, it doesn't work. In giving away the power to print money to the Federal Government without giving ourselves a regular monthly supply, we forgot that we are the source of money.

If we think it is too difficult to get our national government to give us a regular supply of money, we can get our local government to do it.

There are many ways to do this, but the simplest way is through a sales tax. If all exchanges are taxed and this tax income is put in a fund, then the money in this fund can be mailed or otherwise distributed to all the consumers by the local government once a month.

When the money distributed from this fund is spent in the local economy each month it increases because of the principle of compound interest.

Renewal of the Money System

I've tried to write about this before. It is the idea on which Prosperity International was based. As far as I know it has never been expressed before in print. I keep working at simpler and clearer ways of expressing it. This is another attempt.

We are the source of the money system. Money is printed by us. In order for the money system to work we have to distribute to every person in the economy a supply of money. To keep the money system working we have to distribute a supply of money to every person in the economy regularly. The money system must experience renewal. We must resurrect our responsibility for the money system which we have delegated to the Federal government and use it more rationally.

We have permitted our money system to be used without much intelligent control from us, the authors of it. We must realize that money is our servant, not our master. Money has traditionally been used by one person or group to gain power over others and mainly it is used today with short sighted ignorance.

Money is a means of exchange. Money is not wealth, it is a means of exchanging wealth. Wealth is the ideas, goods and services that we produce. Without wealth money would be useless because there would be nothing to buy. Obviously the regular distribution of money to everyone should be related to the total value of the goods and services we are producing. We, the producers, the distributors, and the consumers of wealth are the source of money. We invented and use money for the purpose of facilitating the exchange of the ideas, goods and services that we create. Money works, it is a wonderful invention, but it only works properly when we, the creators of it, the printers of it, give ourselves a regular supply so we can stay in the money game.

This principle was practiced in some cultures who evolved their money system in a more conscious way. The U.S. money system was not evolved rationally by a person or group who understood what money was. I have looked in ancient as well as modern literature about money and never found an adequate discussion of what money is and how a money system is supposed to work. So I decided to meditate on it until I separated the myth from the reality so I could put justice into money—common sense.

The purpose of producing ideas, goods and services is not to earn money. The purpose in nature of producing ideas, goods and services is to have the ideas, goods and services to consume or enjoy. When we produce more ideas, goods and services than we can use ourselves we share them with other people. However, some people produce ideas, goods and services not for the purpose of consuming them themselves, but rather because they have the ability to produce them. In other words, a complex economy with a money system permits specialization to the point where people no longer have to produce for their own needs. They can produce for many reasons. People produce for artistic reasons. They produce for the purpose of accumulating larger bank balances. People produce sometimes for survival but the self-sufficient person who lives directly off the land is rare. In fact, to be self-sufficient means to farm your own food, to make your own clothes and shelter without using any tools produced by other people. Do you have the ability to make your own matches?

The only people I know who are self-sufficient by these definitions are yogi masters like Babaji. Some of them don't need to farm, they can materialize their food directly out of infinite being. Some yogies don't need to eat. Therefore the Republican ideal of economic self sufficiency is a myth in this country. To distribute ideas, goods and services on the basis of some mythical claim to self suffiency is ridiculous. Money is now a necessity in the mind of the average person in order to function conveniently in the U.S. civilization. In our complex economy we are interdependent.

Cars, telephones, governments, indoor plumbing, and central heating systems are inconceivable without a money system. Is this true? To most people it is true. But the real truth is that if everyone used their creativity and productivity out of divine motivation, energy, and love because they enjoyed the self expression and satisfaction of accomplishment, then money would not be necessary. it is a great evil to value money too highly and to be motivated by it without thinking deeply on what we are doing for it. It doesn't take much thought to realize that cars, phones, etc. are not created by money. They are created by people out of the natural resources of the earth, air, water and fire.

Money is a method we have used to distribute our production, but it doesn't work very good when the consumers don't have enough to purchase what is produced. It is appropriate to distribute and use everything that we produce if it is a good product or service and if the production does not involve ruining natural resources or destructive side effects like pollution. Obviously, to use all the nuclear bombs we have produced would be ridiculous. It is also ridiculous to cause people to get sick in order to use all the medicine and hospital equipment that has been produced.

What about food? It is ridiculous to have to consume all the food that we produce. Of course, but in an economy based on abundance, there would be nothing to keep us from exporting our over-production to the rest of the world who would like to use it. Not only food, all kinds of things. This abundant giving may not be enough to prevent war, but it doesn't hurt, except when we export arms and destructive products.

In regard to war, if armament workers had personal prosperity and a regular cash flow, their hunger and insecurity would not be the cause of them working in a defense plant producing the instruments of death.

Now we get a supply of money by producing something and trading it for money or trading our labor for money. But to get the point of being the source of money you have to remember that one time there was none. An individual created some and sold it to others. In most countries the person with the gold mine had a monopoly on money and traded it for everyone's wealth. Then when other people got some gold people used the gold as a means of exchange to trade with anybody.

But what if the people who like to buy our production have no money. Therefore, it is essential for everyone to have a supply of money for the economy to work as it should. Everyone has an abundance of money, then the production, distribution and consumption works, if not, then production is not validated and it stops.

In reality, ideas, goods and services are presently distributed on the basis of an individual's ability to win the money game and personal preference. Receiving government sponsored welfare is included in the concept of winning the money game.

In my opinion it is necessary at this time to design new ways of distributing money. Since we have created a government to print our money for us it is logical to have this government mail every person who participates in the economy a regular supply of money. Or it could be picked up at our local bank or automatically credited to our account. To do this would reduce misery, crime and injustice in our society. To do this would enable the people in our economy to realize more of their potential as human beings as well as in the realm of financial success. It would take the emphasis of work off of money and on value and satisfaction. To give everyone a regular supply of money would have a tendency to stimulate a more universal attitude of abundance, although it must be remembered that ultimately prosperity is an inside job.

As a person, as a consumer, as a producer and participant in the economy, you deserve a regular supply of money. It is your divine right. It is us, the producers of wealth, who have the right to print money to facilitate our exchanges. We have the natural right to print a supply for ourselves regularly and to have it distributed in appropriate amounts to everyone equally in a way that contributes to the self esteem of people and to the health of the economy. If this principle of regularly distributing the money supply is logical, just and honorable, then we have the practical problem of how to sell this principle to the U.S. government which as the printer of U.S. currency is the proper agency to implement it.

We can start by printing copies of this letter and mail them to our congressmen. It is also necessary to distribute copies of this idea to everyone you know, to discuss it with them, and to start building consciousness of these simple thoughts to everyone in your environment. Someone also must write the ideas into the form of legislation in the form that can be introduced in congress. If your congressman doesn't do this as a result of your letter perhaps you will need to follow up your letter with a personal interview in order to motivate your congressman to do this. If you aren't willing to back up these thoughts with political action it will remain just a nice idea forever. I suggest that you reread the chapter on New Age Politics and Economics in *Rebirthing in the New Age*.

I'd like some feedback on these ideas. Ask me questions, argue, whatever. Help me develop these ideas. If I can make them clear to you, maybe we can get them into a form that can be sold.

You are the source of your money system! Are you taking responsibility for this fact?

9 New Age Politics and Economics by Leonard Orr

To be successful, democracy must be firmly grounded in a common sense of personal responsibility for society's welfare and in having a high percentage of the populace actively participating in government. As more and more individuals become enlightened, a permanent grassroots political organization could solve practical problems more efficiently and bring about the infusion of spiritual enlightenment throughout our society. Such an organization could tap the Infinite Intelligence of the entire population for the benefit of all. Innovations of neighborhood representatives and political district councils could turn the political system into a living university that is attached to the real world.

The Psychology of Self-Government

The right to self-government derives from the idea that the whole of Being is present at every point in time and space, and therefore in every individual's mind; that each individual has the right and responsibility to rule his or her own mind, body, and environment. Each person is also responsible for the quality of interaction with other individuals. The basic idea of government is that individuals relate for mutual benefit to accomplish certain objectives that can be more efficiently achieved in relationship than separately. Why hasn't democracy worked? From the viewpoint of the psychology of self-government, Leonard offers two possible explanations.

The first has to do with the parental disapproval syndrome. Parents unwittingly invalidate their children's divine authority, initiative and creativity. The children become addicted to following instructions to get love and, when they grow up, automatically look around for someone to give them permission or tell them how to run their lives. Self-government goes out the window. Groups of enlightened individuals have established democracies from time to time in human history and the parental disapproval syndrome causes them to evolve back into dictatorships. People are unwilling to govern themselves because on a deep emotional level they have been conditioned to believe that they don't really have the right.

Today we have what we might call a dictatorship of the bureaucracy, which may be the worst of all, because everyone is running around carrying out instructions that nobody started and that nobody can change. So there is a maze of helplessness. It is children taking out their suppressed hostility towards their parents on other children who are helpless to defend themselves. It is only possible to win by realizing that you are the source of government and therefore the source of bureaucracy. The dictatorship of the bureaucracy will only be defeated as individuals operate from their own divine authority.

The virtue of the contemporary American situation is that the U. S. Constitution spelled out basic divine rights clearly enough to intimidate the helpless bureaucrats. The purpose of the bureaucracy is to serve the individual. If this is kept clearly in mind, one individual can make it true for himself in spite of the confusion in his environment.

New age thinking is reviving the respect of the individual for his or her own authority and divine rights. Our present society has many spiritual giants, as well as helpless psychological dependents. There already may be enough self-sufficient individuals to make democracy work. So all that is needed is reform in the political structure that will make it possible for these spiritual giants to manifest and to raise the level of government to the point where democracy can function successfully.

Our democracy is a Republican democracy. Pure democracy involves everyone in all the decisions. Republican democracy is delegating some of the decisions to individuals that are elected by everyone. The types of decisions that our elected representatives are authorized to make are defined by the constitution that defines each body of representatives. The principle of constitutional government is to limit the power of governmental bodies so that they serve the citizenry. In other words, in democracy, the government is ruled by the people. The individual is supreme authority. When the representatives exceed their constitutional powers, the electorate has to replace them.

In order for our democratic political structure to be functional, the ratio of representation must be adequate to make quality communication possible between the electorate and the representatives. The electorate has to have enough knowledge of the particular decision of its representatives to judge the worthiness of their constitutional performance. When the ratio of representation becomes too large, quality of communication, and therefore of democracy, declines.

The contemporary manifestation of the psychological problem of democracy is that our citizens act like someone else controls the representatives, the way they were elected, and the ratio of representation, instead of themselves. The citizens forget that they *are* the government, and wait helplessly for their elected representatives to reform government and solve the problems. The elected representatives are waiting for the citizens. So everybody sits around complaining and nobody solves the problems. (The elected representatives only have as much divine authority as the people who elect them!)

Obviously the only solution is for enlightened individuals who are successfully ruling their own lives to take over the positions of authority and use them to educate the citizenry in their own spiritual enlightenment. Until government becomes the instrument of spiritual aristocracy, the situation is hopeless. The central issue is whether or not spiritually enlightened individuals participate or run for cover!

The second explanation of what is wrong with the psychology of our nation and of western culture is religious in nature. The issue of physical death illustrates it more clearly than anything. The Judeo-Christian religions have traditionally affirmed that physical death is beyond our control. This belief inevitably keeps *life* beyond our control. It comes out of a theology that God is outside ourselves. As long as people believe that God is outside themselves, then the power of government will be outside themselves. *The original sin is to believe that you are not God.* If you are not God, you will forever cop out when it comes to self-government. This might be called a "religious inferiority complex."

As long as people believe that God is outside of human beings and has the power to murder them arbitrarily for his own reasons, then governments will reflect this belief. Crime, murder and war comes out of this belief in such a capricious God. Crime, capital punishment, murder and war are not sociological problems, but individuals misbehaving as a protest for having their divinity invalidated. Divine beings express divine love, harmony and wisdom in their behavior. *The only solution to the problems of the world is the exaltation of personal divinity.*

The new age thought is that the universe is waiting for the divine man and woman and that the triumph of the spiritual aristocracy is inevitable. This should be obvious to all thinking persons. (For example, people who believe in war will get together and kill each other.) Polluters that are successful will destroy themselves when their environment no longer supports them. Therefore, it is obvious that only the wise and self-sufficient will survive. And if a person does not have enough spiritual enlightenment to believe in physical immortality, then he or she will be destroyed by his or her own mind.

Some people still think that physical immortality is difficult to achieve, or irrelevant and esoteric. The truth is that it is the foundation of spiritual enlightenment. It is the *first step,* not the last step! If you can't take responsibility for the destiny of your physical body, which you can see, then taking responsibility for your soul, which you can't see, is hopeless. The wise men once said that if you can't master physical things, then no one will trust you with the true riches of the soul. If the destiny of your physical body is uncertain, so is the spiritual destiny of your soul. If you don't take responsibility for the destiny and welfare of your physical body, why should you take responsibility for your environment? Ecology is pointless without physical immortality. Democracy will keep dying as long as people die. If you are not willing to take responsibility for the destiny of your body, neither will you be willing to take responsibility for the destiny of your nation or the planet.

The Ratio of Representation

The key to republican democracy is the ratio of representation. Leonard's conclusion is that, for democracy to work structurally, a minimum ratio of representation of 1 to 1,000 is required. It is impractical to expect one person to adequately represent the political concepts of more than a thousand people. *It may be unrealistic for a person to satisfactorily represent ten others!* (Some married couples have difficulty representing the views of their partners accurately.) This defines the problem of the ratio of representation.

A representative has the responsibility of speaking for people he or she represents. The question is: how many people is the optimum number for one person to represent in a meaningful manner politically? In the average American city today, the ratio of representation is 1 to 100,000 people. On the county, state and national basis, the ratio of representation may be one to a million and a half! In other words, in Los Angeles County, for example, the County Supervisor is expected to represent a million and a half people. The emperors of history's greatest empires never represented that many people, and yet we have that kind of ridiculous situation in a country that claims to be a democracy.

What has happened to the minds of the people who are raised in the public schools that are supposed to teach democracy and yet have not figured out the obvious contradictions or corrected them? How can seven million people in the county of Los Angeles ignore the political hypocracy that they are living in? An ideal functional representation unit is probably one hundred people. Since this is an unrealistic goal for large cities in the immediate future, Leonard recommends that we shoot for an immediate reform of 1 to 1,000.

Let's take a look at the immediate implications of this reform in our present political structure. Most major cities have voting precincts that have a voter registration of four to five hundred and a total population of a thousand. Voter precincts are good units to use for neighborhood organization because they are clearly defined, so let's call this political reform of the ratio of representation "neighborhood representation" or "precinct representation."

You can't wait for the government to solve the problem and you can't wait for your neighbor to solve the problem. *You* have to solve the problem. If you are reading this and you understand it, then obviously God has already appointed you to be the Savior and hero or heroine of this nation.

So the goal is to organize your political precinct into an effective neighborhood organization. (If you are not enlightened when you start this project, you will be when you finish it.) The foundation of the neighborhood organization is a monthly town meeting in which human concerns of all individuals in the neighborhood are discussed. If there were only one spiritually enlightened person in the neighborhood, that town meeting would contain the element of self-improvement, and everyone would have an opportunity to know the truth about life.

Next, the neighborhood organization must have an elected representative who functions in district associations for each political district. In other words, there would be a counsel of neighborhood representatives for the city council district that would meet with the city council. There would be another council of neighborhood representatives who would meet with the county's elected officials once a month. There would be another council of neighborhood representatives to meet with the State Assemblymen once each month. And finally, a council of neighborhood representatives in each Congressional District to meet with the Congressmen.

This means that the neighborhood representative would attend five meetings a month: with the neighborhood town meeting; with the City Councilmen; with the County Supervisor; with the State Assemblymen; and with the Congressmen. He would supply the average citizen with a monthly cycle of communications with each level of government.

The implications of this simple reform for the quality of life in our existing society are infinite. What this application of the ratio of representation principle would create is a sociological pyramid. A pyramid has graduated geometric progression from bottom to top. A republican democracy must have similar graduated levels of representation, each level being directly responsible to its contingency of individual citizens, which acknowledges a dependency of the top on the base.

The manner in which this improvement in political structure transforms the electoral process, the contemporary problems of education, senior citizens, child development, ecology, utilization of natural resources, space travel, economics, social and political issues, is too large a subject to describe adequately in this book. Therefore, we suggest you read *How to Make Democracy Work,* a book on grassroots politics by Leonard, available at all Theta centers.

The ratio of representation must also be applied to international politics. The United Nations is a good idea but it can't be called a democratic body until there is a house of representatives at the United Nations that truly represents the citizens of the world.

The network of neighborhood representation, together with district councils, becomes an interpenetrating communication system for a whole society that functions like a living university. This university expands the consciousness of the individual and as the consciousness of the individual becomes more enlightened, the university produces more wonderful results in our society. So the psychology of self-government and the political structure with an adequate ration of representation serve each other.

The ultimate model for the ratio of representation is as ancient as Moses and is clearly spelled out in Exodus 18 of the Protestant Bible.

In a sense, politics is the ultimate spiritual work. Your neighbor who works with you today may be your political enemy working against you tomorrow on a different issue! Obviously, this is the greatest test for love. It stretches your wisdom and builds character. In politics, you can't run away or quit because it affects your life whether you like it or not. When you take responsibility in your neighborhood, you are forced to live the brotherhood of man and the fatherhood of God on the most practical level. If spiritual enlightenment doesn't lead to political participation, it is impractical if not worthless.

It is up to you to make these ideas work; the only way you will ever solve the problems of the world is to solve them in your neighborhood. The wisdom and riches of the President will not free your neighbor from suffering. If you are enlightened, then you are the teacher of truth, the instrument of deliverance for your neighbors. It is time for spiritual people to get off Cloud Nine and practice the good neighbor policy literally by loving real physical next door neighbors verbally and materially.

Citizen's Prosperity Dividend Fund

It is ridiculous to profess to be spiritually enlightened and not take responsibility for political and economic problems. Taxes proves the point dramatically. The average person has 20 to 30 percent of his or her paycheck withheld by the government for income taxes, which means that the average person works a day and a half or more out of every week for the Federal Government—whether he likes it or not. The truth is that if you are not active in politics, you are a slave. If you are not controlling your public servants, then you automatically become a servant of government. The following idea is a simple, direct way of eliminating this slavery.

The three foundations of macroeconomics are imagination, labor and consumption. Distribution is the link between labor and consumption; "labor" includes entrepreneurs and management. Imagination has been applied more to production than to distribution and consumption. What is necessary is to transform the public cash flow at a basic level. This basic transformation will distribute the wealth more efficiently and equitably, and free the productive energy and imagination of both entrepreneurs and workers. It will stimulate the opportunity and prosperity of both consumers and businesses.

The least-honored factor in traditional macroeconomic theory is the customer. Production is worthless without consumption. Consumers must have money in order to purchase the production. Except for spotty social welfare programs, no organic instrument has been established in our economy to flow the cash back to the consumer so that the consumer can keep the producer in business. There is a bit of spiritual genius in this reform that will produce a high degree of integrity in our economic system that may not be seen by the casual thinker. It is this: the concept of a citizen's prosperity fund creates a quantity of economic freedom for the average person that stimulates the greatest of all economic values—*love of work* and *work of love.*

When the masses are financially independent, mountains of worthless junk are not as likely to be produced. When the laborer is financially independent, and not forced to work out of necessity, then he or she becomes more ethical about the quality of work he or she is willing to do.

Obviously it doesn't matter how much money consumers have if there are not goods and services to consume. Economic freedom and financial independence cannot eliminate labor, but economic freedom will restore the holiness and true value of manual labor. Leonard has three important conclusions:

1. Manual labor is essential to mental and physical health. This is more true for the rich than the poor.
2. Rich people work harder than poor people because they love their work.

3. In fact, most people (both rich and poor) are not motivated by money but by habit. Therefore, regardless of macro-economic changes in the cash flow, for the benefit of the average citizen, things will go on much as they are. This leads to the conclusion that education and not money is the only redeemer.

Citizens' Prosperity Fund

The purpose of the Citizen's Prosperity Fund is to expand prosperity consciousness, to stimulate personal creativity, to stimulate the local and world economy through the "multiplier effect," and to redistribute cash flow more equitably to the poor.

All human wealth is created by the human mind. Money and the money system were created to serve people, not to inhibit them. There are four basic laws to the money system:

1. Earning or Production   2. Spending or Exchange
3. Saving   4. Investing

1. Earning or Production—All human production comes out of human imagination.
2. Spending—Exchanging production increases the quality and quantity of human wealth in the world.
3. Saving—Accumulating surpluses that serve appropriate personal purposes facilitates wealth.
4. Investing—Using past production to increase present and future production.

The Prosperity Fund is based on the conclusion that the spending law is the most neglected one in modern economical systems. The citizens behind the Fund believe that consumer cash flow is a valuable element to think about. The citizens involved in Prosperity International believe that education, imagination and practical effort are the cures of money problems. But we also believe that every consumer has a natural right to a regular personal cash flow as a necessary element to make the money system work with optimum justice and efficiency. We believe a regular personal cash flow for everyone keeps everybody in the game playing at a higher level of self esteem, freedom and personal morality, and that balancing the spending law through this program will enrich humanity spiritually, mentally, physically, socially and economically.

The basic idea of the Prosperity Fund is to establish a bank account to be filled with money which is to be distributed equally in monthly payments to all residents in a defined geographical territory. Initially, the Fund is filled by voluntary contributions from successful individuals and businesses, but it is hoped that when the Fund idea gains wide acceptance, it will become an element in governmental budgets.

The Prosperity Fund is administered by a committee of local citizens who prefer to remain anonymous for humanitarian reasons. For further information, contact Prosperity International.

It may be helpful in the administration and communication of this program to have a neighborhood coordinator for every 10-25 residents. If you are willing to serve your community in this way, please check the box on the card by the word "volunteer."

This is a strictly voluntary program. It implies no obligation in any way for either givers or receivers nor members of the committee. Any participant may withdraw at any time without notice.

This program is intended to be a worthy experiment in prosperity education. Obviously, it is not a substitute for working since there would be nothing to buy if nobody produced. Its function is to redistribute money, goods and services more justly and efficiently, to free human imagination and resources.

The program is based on the four laws of wealth that were originally taught by Leonard Orr through the famous Money Seminar. It seems to be a simple way of applying the principles of prosperity presented in the Money Seminar to our community. The basic principles of the Money Seminar are that all human wealth is created by the human mind and that imagination, education and practical effort can solve any financial problem. Money is created by humans to encourage production by making the exchanging process more convenient. Everyone can develop a prosperity consciousness and be successful financially.

The four laws of wealth are:

1. Earning or Production
2. Spending or Exchanging
3. Saving
4. Investing

More information on the four laws of wealth can be received from Prosperity International.

This idea can be initiated and implemented by anyone simply by forming a local prosperity fund that mails out dividends regularly.

1. Any person or business can establish the fund by contributing voluntarily 1 percent of their income, or whatever, into the fund monthly.
2. The fund mails out the money equally to all residents.
3. Labor on the fund is donated and the fund can be supervised by local government.
4. Some benefits of this program:
   - Redistributes wealth.
   - Increases cash flow of the poor.
   - Simulates local, national and world economies.
   - Gives people a subsidy income between jobs.
   - Increases quality of work decision.
   - Frees people for creative pursuits.
   - Creates more opportunity for self-improvement.
   - Not based on prejudice and bureaucracy.
5. Ideas to make it work better:
   - The dividend check is void if not cashed within 30 days.

- Might be better to distribute cash through neighborhood representatives to save paper and labor.
6. Any corruption should never be a crime, because money is not worth freedom and any damage to the system can be corrected in 30 days. It's only money. The real production and imagination that the system stimulates is the real value.
7. The most efficient kind of charity I can think of.
8. You can start this project in your community by picking a geographical territory and registering people and businesses to participate. Since it is a sound program, it grows rapidly.
9. A few forward-thinking thoughts:
   - It is up to the banks to determine that the committee is legitimate until local government takes it on. You might check to make sure before participating.
   - It may be better to use scrip rather than bank checks in some cases.
   - It may be better to use cash than either scrip or checks since it saves paper, natural resources and processing.
   - It may be better to distribute the money through neighborhood coordinators rather than the mails.

If you would like to support the spread of this program worldwide, send your contributions to:

Citizens Prosperity Fund
Prosperity International
P.O. Box 234
Sierraville, CA 96126
(916) 994-8984 or (916) 994-3677

Send for related information. Speakers available.

Here is a sample letter to prospective participants in the citizen's prosperity fund:

Dear Resident,

This money was donated by individuals who are financially successful. Financial success is good for us; it made us more generous, more loving and more creative. We desire everyone to have a perpetual guaranteed income. This voluntary community fund is the best idea we could think of to share our wealth.

This fund can provide you with a perpetual income if local merchants and other wealthy persons also make contributions to this fund on a monthly basis. Merchants who contribute 1 percent of their monthly gross income will be mentioned when you receive your check so that you can prosper them and increase their participation. This idea can stimulate jobs and creativity by increasing the cash flow in our local economy.

The idea behind this fund will work if you are willing to receive the check and spend it immediately. Everyone is welcome to give into the fund 1 percent of personal income. It is fun to participate in your local economy in this way and see if what you give is more than what you receive.

The principles of this prosperity program contain the secret of wealth. They are applied by every bank, common stock corporation and wealthy individuals. Finally, someone has figured out a realistic way to apply them to the poor and to every common person who is willing to prosper. The basic principle is the spiritual truth that makes money work. The principle of money itself—exchange by faith.

It may be helpful in the administration and communication of this program to have a neighborhood coordinator for every 10–25 residents. If you are willing to serve your community in this way, please check the box on the card by the word "volunteer."

The fund is administered by a committee of local citizens who prefer to remain anonymous for humanitarian reasons. For further information, contact your village clerk or bank.

This is a strictly voluntary program. It implies no obligation in any way for either givers or receivers nor members of the committee. Any participant may withdraw at any time without notice. This program is intended to be a worthy experiment in prosperity education.

Obviously, this program is not a substitute for working since there would be nothing to buy if nobody produces. Its function is to redistribute money, goods and services more justly and efficiently, to free human imagination and resources.

You are welcome to receive more information about this program by attending a Money Seminar free (even though it has a price published in our publicity). This program seems to be a simple way of applying the principles of prosperity presented in the Money Seminar to our community.

Taxes and Profits

Here is a simple idea that can eliminate poverty completely and also eliminate taxes as a burden! The idea is, essentially, to make our government a business corporation and to make all citizens stockholders. Every citizen becomes financially independent on dividends, as a shareholder in the total economy. This tax reform will take three essential steps.

First, in your mind at least, eliminate all taxes: income, corporate, sales, business, property, estate, and any other kinds— which of course eliminates the bureaucracies that collect them. Then establish only three kinds of taxation.

(1) Sales tax on all consumer goods and services because it is based on exchanging production. This is the best of all forms of taxation as long as it is combined with the dividend system described below.

(2) A straight income tax of 1 percent. The present graduated systems are based on false and totally illogical premises and are completely obsolete and unfair to everyone. This should be collected morally, not legally. One percent may seem small, but as you will soon see, it is more than enough.

(3) A social welfare tax which is contributed voluntarily. This would be given out of income or net worth. It replaces property taxes, estate taxes and a few others.

These tax methods are based on the solid principle of "no taxation without representation." Only people (who are called consumers economically) can have representation: therefore only people can be taxed. All present corporation taxes, for example, are built into the price of the product and the consumer-citizen ends up paying them anyway. Why not place them out into the open as a sales tax so we can vote on them? The tyranny of the present tax situation is unspeakably oppressive and these are very rational changes.

The second step is to establish one taxing agency which is directly controlled by a vote of the people. This one agency collects all taxes and distributes the government's portion equitably among the various levels of government. For example, 40 percent of tax income is paid to city government, 30 percent to the county, 20 percent to the state, and 10 percent to the Federal Government. This formula is only a suggested one, but whatever the percentages are, they can be adjusted annually by a vote of the people. We, the people, are paying the taxes to our government for our purposes and it is time that we demonstrated our control over this area in an intelligent, orderly way.

The final step is to establish a consumer's dividend fund which is mailed equally to all citizens on at least a monthly basis. It is an inversion of the graduated income tax and it fulfills the original purpose of the graduated system. All tax income is divided into two portions. For example, 50 percent of the income is allocated to government budgets and the other 50 percent is paid to the consumer dividend fund. The dividend fund functions as a group savings account which is invested in our consumer economy to yield future profits. The best place to invest this dividend fund is to divide it up and mail it to consumers equally as a monthly dividend on the total cash flow of all business in the nation. This monthly dividend check gives all citizens a guaranteed monthly income that eliminates hardcore proverty and that produces a good measure of economic freedom to the individual. It also supplies a guaranteed cash flow in the local economy and, for all practical purposes, eliminates major depressions or recessions for the nation. This dividend fund would eliminate the major corruptions and inequities of our present social welfare systems as well as the inequities of the present system of taxation.

In the American capitalistic system, laborers agree to accept certain wages even though they may be disproportionate to the amount of profits their work actually produces. This is just and fair because the entrepreneur deserves a great reward for the creativity and risk he takes in assuming his role in our economy. The dividend fund system of taxation balances out this labor contribution and increases personal economic freedom in a way that benefits all concerned. This inequity in profits is partially corrected by some companies through profit-sharing programs. It can only be corrected totally by a national profit-sharing program. Profit incentives for both laborer and entrepreneur are being strangled by present tax laws.

Please understand the nature of profit. Basically, profit is created by the arbitrary fiat of the individual producer or businessman. A retailer, for example, purchases an item at one price and sells it at a higher price. He decides how much profit he shall receive, subject to the consumer's veto. Then he spends his profit and thereby permits the next person to profit. All taxes are actual ly profit that is created in the economy for the government. Taxes are profits from the flow of wealth in our economy for the pur pose of community welfare. The individual citizen, who is the owner of the government, has the moral and economic right to a direct percentage of these profits. This concept can be applied to a neighborhood Chamber of Commerce or a city government, as well as on a county, state, or federal level.

The four laws of wealth: (production, spending, saving and investing) are the laws by which every bank, savings and loan, successful corporation, and wealthy individual have achieved success. It is time that we applied these same laws to ourselves as a total society to eliminate poverty and make all of us financially independent. Actually, stock corporations and savings and loan associations have already done this with their small societies. Doing it as a nation puts our government (us) in a stronger financial position.

If everyone is financially independent, who is going to do the work? Ask yourself: Who are the greatest producers now? They are those people who are already financially independent. Financial independence doesn't prevent people from working, rather it takes the lid off their energy and their creative potential. Wealthy people love to work more than anyone because they are free to choose what they do. Entrepreneurs and capitalists don't work to make a living—they know that work is love made visible.

The tax reforms here suggested unleash the profit motive and set men free to produce. Our economy has never been endangered by too many wealthy people. On the contrary, it has been stifled when consumers lack money to purchase our production. The problem of our people will never be production of wealth. It has always been the distribution of wealth.

The two foundations of economics are production and distribution. The American economy has traditionally overproduced in every category. The bottleneck in our economy has traditionally been inequitable distribution of goods and services. The key to this bottleneck is the distribution of money. This dividend concept redistributes the cash flow on a monthly basis in an equitable way so that everyone can stay in the money game. When you think this system through, you will realize that it enables everyone to win.

More New Age Politics

Three good ideas by Leonard Orr:
1. Monthly town meetings on every block.
2. Tax reform by individual initiative.
3. Elected professional neighborhood leaders.

The benefits of grassroots politics are infinite. I could write hundreds of books about implications of neighborhood representation through monthly block meetings. My goal here is to suggest several simple practices that come from the heart of the American tradition. I believe these simple innovations will regenerate the average citizen and rehabilitate a taste of victory. These simple ideas can cure apathy in the average citizen and make him or her a conscious and intelligent participator. My desire is to keep this so brief that people can read it quickly, reproduce it cheaply and use it to spread the ideas rapidly. The three following ideas work together.

IDEA 1. *Have a monthly town meeting on every block or each rural area of 100 people or less.* The monthly block meeting is the key to rehabilitating American republican democracy. Each block meeting must elect a leader in order to make it work. If each block has an *elected* leader, who delivers a monthly newsletter to everybody on the block, reporting on his or her activities, it doesn't matter whether anybody comes to the monthly meetings or not. However, monthly meetings are fun, educational, entertaining and therapeutic. They can also be good for business, and spiritual enlightenment. The most important purpose is to build successful relationships among the people on the block that are filled with peace, understanding and harmony, based in truth, simplicity and love.

Monthly block meetings as the foundation for the pyramid of good government can easily be integrated into our existing political structure by requiring a council meeting for the block leaders for each level of government. In other words, your block leader can meet with your city councilperson, county supervisor, state assemblyperson and congressperson once each month. All elected representatives meet with the council of block leaders for all the blocks in his or her district once each month. This creates a monthly cycle of communication that goes both ways between the voters and their elected officials. This idea is called neighborhood representation. It is the ultimate goal of grassroots politics.

IDEA 2. *Tax reform* by individual initiative. Here is a simple, instantaneous, legal and what could be totally effective personal tax-reform program. This idea can change the whole ridiculous complicated and oppressive tax structure in this country in one year. But it is totally dependent upon your courage and initiative. You must act, don't wait for the other guy. If you act on this idea now and pass it on so will other people. If you aren't good enough to act upon this idea why should you expect other people to do it? The idea is simple. It is based upon your willingness to pay only ten percent of your personal income for taxes each month.

To make the idea work, you divide your ten percent among the existing levels of government that you believe in and mail it monthly to your elected officials for each level of government. I suggest the following formula:

> 2% to block leader
> 2% to city councilperson
> 2% to county supervisor
> 1% to state assemblyperson
> 1% to national congressperson
> 1% to United Nations
> 1% to your favorite fund for community
>   and world betterment
> 10% total monthly tax payments

I suggest that you make out your check to the City of San Francisco, for example, and mail them each month to the city councilperson. Make out your national check to the U.S. Government and mail it to the name of your U.S. Congressperson. In other words, the goal is to make your elected representatives personally responsible to you the voter for the financial success of the government they are supposed to manage. This practice makes them aware of the fact that you desire tax reform and that you desire it now instead of in some distant century of the future.

If this tax personal reform initiative fails, you can deduct whatever you pay during the year from your income taxes at the end of the year. This willingness on your part is important to make this tax reform movement legal. The goal of tax reform is not to destroy the government or make it fail financially, the goal is to make our government financially responsible to us, the taxpayers.

I believe we all desire most of the wonderful services that our governments provide. Who is willing to give up freeways or fire and police protection, for example? It is time to rehabilitate your love and responsibility for government.

There are several other facts that can be helpful to you in making this proposal work:

Fact 1. The IRS has a simple form which would prevent your employer from withholding income taxes from your pay check. Your employer can send this tax reform initiative with the withholding tax reports to the IRS, along with your name and Social Security number.

Fact 2. To change the sales tax system, you can give this personal tax reform document to retail merchants and ask them to include it with their sales tax returns stating on the report the amount of tax that was not collected.

Fact 3. Property tax bills could be returned with this tax reform document and a letter stating that the existing tax rate is not acceptable to you and that you are sending your tax money directly to your elected officials until the government comes up with a system that you like better than the one they are now using.

Fact 4. It is necessary to remember that no one in this country has experienced real republican democracy for over one hundred years. So be patient! If you can build a well-attended block meeting in one year, you are doing very well. People have accumulated a lifetime of frustration about politics. People need lots of practice to express themselves in a practical way. Harmony and agreement about anything may take time. Tax is a hot issue. Proceed with love and patience. Slowliness is holiness.

Fact 5. Obviously, if a few hundred thousand people across the country practiced this tax reform initiative it would be a totally safe and effective way to achieve the desired result of tax reform very rapidly.

Obviously, you will feel safer and more supported if you practice this idea with the people on your block or with your civic or religious group, but the beauty of this idea is that you can do it all by yourself and get results. Like I said, if it doesn't work by the end of the year, you just deduct what you have already paid through this system when you fill out the standard tax forms.

The Declaration of Independence which freed this country from the oppressive taxes of England is the basis of this personal tax reform initiative. The government is our servant, not our master. The U.S. Constitution does not give the government the right to tax us without our consent. The personal tax reform initiative idea puts the principle of renewal into our oppressive tax structures. It can easily spread to a million people in one year.

The IRS is often acused of tactics worse than the British soldiers used in the 1700s. It is time for a New Age American Revolution. Now is the time for enlightened Americans to take responsibility for our own governments.

IDEA 3. *The elected block leader should be a well-paid full-time job.* The elected block leader is a professional citizen. This person is a full-time voter, a professional human being who hopefully is also divine. This person would be a wise and loving person. A person with common sense and a sense of humor. We should elect the best person on the block. This job is for a person who can organize and conduct orderly meetings, who is a counselor and therapist, a friend when in trouble. Kindness and friendship are still among the greatest virtues. The block leader is also a lobbyist for fellow voters. Everyone has lobbyists but the voters these days.

The economics of paying block leaders are simple. A monthly town meeting territory should consist of 50–200 people to be represented by one block leader. Let's use the figure of 100 people, taxpayers or voters. The average person has an income of over $100 per week. The average person has 25 to 50 percent of each week's income withheld for federal income taxes. Therefore if 2 percent goes to the block leader, each person with a $100 per week income on the block pays $2 per week or $8 per month (to save, say, $30 per week or $120 per month). Political apathy costs the average citizen at least two full days of work every week. Apathy costs big money. Most people work half of their lives to support a government they say they don't believe in. Obviously, this is hypocrisy. Paying 10 percent of your income is one half day per week for the government. Paying 50 percent of your income to the government is a form of slavery. Another alternate—if you can find a good person in your neighborhood who is willing to do this job for $100 per week, it only takes $10 per week from ten supportive people to pay a salary.

Obviously it makes good business sense for us the citizens to do this. It seems to me, that it is a practical way to make the brotherhood and sisterhood of humankind at least a possibility. If harmony, spiritual enlightenment, truth, simplicity and love dominate monthly town meetings, we may even become inspired to think about heaven on earth.

To have a full-time elected neighborhood leader on every block is the most effectve way to solve all of our political, social, and economic problems that I can think of. Let's try it, if it doesn't work we can get our neighborhood leaders to abolish the idea.

Three ideas: 1. A monthly town meeting on every block. 2. Tax Reform by individual initiative. 3. Professional elected block leaders—a new career. These are three good ideas that can prevent an infinite amount of trouble and cause an infinite amount of consciousness and happiness. These simple ideas can harness an infinite potential of benefits for every one of us.

Your positive participation is invited.

Your friend and fellow citizen,

Leonard Orr
Box 234
Sierraville, CA 96126
(916) 994-8984 or 994-3677

10 Your Perfect Weight

It is not what you eat that hurts you, it is what you *believe* about what you eat. Your body always obeys the instructions of your mind. It is the instructions you give to food that matter. A physical technique for losing weight works because your mind believes it. A study was done on people who were weighing precisely their desirable weight and it was found that they all could eat anything they wanted without concern or worry. They could do this because they believed that they could eat anything without getting fat. "I never gain weight," they would say or "I never worry about what I eat." *Actually, we are nourished by the Light of God, not by food.* There are people who have not eaten for twenty-five years. Therese Newman is one of them. And there are many other saints you can read about who can do this. We actually met one in India so I was finally able to verify this fact.

When people at Leonard's weight seminar are asked what they feel is the real cause of their overweight, they cite anxiety, sexual deprivation, nerves, food, boredom, self-hate, self-pity, glands, lack of exercise, laziness, loneliness, lack of fulfillment, lack of affection, rebellion, depression, etc.

How scientific are weight problems? According to science, you can only have one cause for a particular condition. If sexual deprivation caused weight problems then everybody who was sexually deprived would be overweight. And if nerves caused overweight, then everybody who was nervous would be overweight. If food caused weight problems, then everybody who eats a lot would have a weight problem, and that is not true either. Everybody who is bored would have a weight problem if there is a cause-and-effect relationship; everybody who felt self-hate or self-pity would have a weight problem if that really caused overweight. If glands were the problem, then it would be impossible to lose weight unless you changed your glands; most people who do cure their weight problem don't do it with glandular treatment.

From time to time we have people come to the weight seminar who have an underweight problem. When they are asked to make a list of the causes of their underweight, the list comes out the same as the list made by overweight people!

Attitude and belief are the common denominators of all the causes of obesity. In other words, what causes you to be overweight is what you believe. Everybody who has a weight problem believes that *something* is causing it. Well, the cause that produces results (i.e., the weight problem) 100 percent of the time is *thought*. What you think is always involved. Anybody who has dieted knows that dieting does not produce permanent results unless one were to diet from negative thought about his body! If you diet from negative thoughts about your body, then it would produce permanent results. What you need to do is to abstain from negative thoughts and feast on positive thoughts! This will produce permanent results characterized by beauty, health and joy.

One man came to a weight seminar wanting to lose ten pounds. We didn't see him again until he came to a money seminar eight months later. He told us that he had only been able to remember two affirmations from the weight seminar, but by the end of the week he had lost ten pounds and never gained it back. The two affirmations were: "Everything I eat turns to health and beauty" and "My body automatically processes whatever food I eat to maintain my perfect weight of _____." All we had done at that seminar was to sit around and design affirmations for every one of the causes people listed, changing each from a weight problem to a weight solution. The impact of doing that for four hours one night just melted the weight right off his body.

At another weight seminar we tried the "eating experiment"; together we made a shopping list of all our favorite foods, then sent a committee out at one of the breaks to buy them all. So we sat around eating pizza, ice cream, cheese cake, baklava, enchiladas, chocolate chip cookies, hamburgers, pastries and fig bars for the rest of the seminar. Everyone tried to get the maximum amount of pleasure, eating anything as long as they enjoyed it. The idea was to keep from going unconscious while enjoying oneself. People found they had a lot of difficulty enjoying their favorite foods! The long-term results varied. One man lost fifteen pounds in the next three days! Other people developed more consciousness and discipline about their food.

The affirmations principle has the power to solve all weight problems. It is important to note that all affirmations work, including the one that says "Affirmations don't work." If you work with the affirmations in this chapter, they will lead you to your *personal law* on weight. Everyone has a dominant consciousness factor, or personal law, in regard to any physical or psychological condition. A personal law is formed over years, and it might take a year to break it. But you will never break it if you don't start.

Most of us have tried dieting and found that it doesn't really work. However, once you use psychological principles to lose weight, there is a role that dieting can play. At the beginning you can diet or fast in order to "prime the pump." While we are working with affirmations and convincing your mind that your thoughts control the situation, dieting kind of seduces your subconscious into believing the new concepts. It gives them greater strength. What you will notice is that if you diet without suggestion, you will go back to the same place and if you diet with suggestion, you will never go back to the same place. You may go halfway back. If you only go halfway back each time you diet, pretty soon you will be right where you want to be. On the other hand, if your mind is willing to accept weight loss without dieting, then you can skip dieting altogether!

The most important affirmation is this one: "I like my body. The more I like it the more lovable it becomes." That is really powerful because the basic law of the mind is the law of increase. Whatever you concentrate upon increases. The basic dynamic in psychosomatic principles is that your body totally obeys you. If you say "My finger is going to bend," your finger will obey you every time. Your finger will stay straight if you command it to stay straight. Your body has no choice but to obey you! Weight problems, then, are obviously created by your mind and your body follows your instructions—so the first objective in changing your body is to change your mind.

One of the ways you can do that is by writing affirmations. Write each of them ten or twenty times a day (trust your intuitive sense about which ones are the most valuable). The first one is, "I like my body." If you say "I don't like my body," then your body has to do whatever you *don't* want it to do in order to please you! The body will go on getting heavier and heavier . . . See the paradox? You must totally accept the idea that your body is pleasing you and that you love your body. You *can* love your body for being overweight because it is being obedient to your mind. But that same obedience can produce different results.

In regard to food, the basic affirmation is, "My body automatically processes whatever food I eat to maintain my perfect weight." If you have been saying that your body doesn't cooperate with you, then your perfect weight is non-cooperation. If you write out the affirmation and, each time, write your emotional reaction to it on the side, your reactions will eventually lead you to everything in your subconsious. Then your natural truth will shine uninhibitedly. The affirmation principle is a way of totally purging your mind.

The next affirmation is, "My perfect weight is _____." Write in your absolutely perfect weight, not an intermediate goal. Your mind will produce whatever you put in that affirmation. If you put down an intermediate goal, you will produce the intermediate goal and then you will have to reprogram your mind to a lower goal. So affirm your absolutely perfect weight and your absolutely perfect dimensions, because that is what you will get.

Another good affirmation about food is, "Everything I eat turns to health and beauty." There are all kinds of variations, like, "Everything I put into my mouth is good for me." Jesus said, for example, that it is not what you eat that hurts you, it is what you believe about what you eat that hurts you. That is why people who go on diets without protein *can* do fine if they believe that you don't need protein to exist. People used to eat fat to get thin, remember? Remember the polyunsaturated fats theory? Leonard once had a health food store, and people came in to buy fat capsules. It worked for some people and it didn't work for other people, according to their belief. The people it didn't work for would come in and say, "Well, I am going to try this, but I don't think it is going to work." They would come back feeling helpless and say, "Nothing can solve my problem." That is an affirmation; the body will obey such a command and nothing will happen. Leonard has at least two friends who have gone without food or water for sixty days or more with no harm to themselves.

There was one woman who came to a weight seminar who weighed about three hundred pounds. We found out that her grandparents died of tuberculosis and they were emaciated when they died. The family tradition was, "You will be healthy if you have a few extra pounds!" But they never told her how many extra pounds was enough. So she kept adding extra pounds—for her it was a survival mechanism. If she had a few extra pounds she wouldn't die, but if she lost weight she was in danger of dying, or so her mind had it. Obviously, nothing she ever tried worked because losing weight meant death to her.

Our parents told us that if we didn't eat, something terrible would happen to us. Food is connected to illness and death. And also, probably one of the things we were certain about getting love for, getting praise for, was cleaning our plate. As a result, whenever we feel insecure or depressed we go back to that activity that brought us love as children: cleaning up our plates. So food is all tied up with love because people cleaned up their plate to get approval.

It is necessary to realize that you don't have to eat at all in order to maintain health and that you can eat only every other day. In fact, that would be a valuable form of discipline: Eat only every other day for a week and notice the "numbers" you run on yourself when you are doing that. The reason you often get a headache when you feel you have to eat something is due to the command programmed in you that if you don't eat, something terrible will happen.

This is really a powerful technique. Try it! Get out your fine china, fine silverware, add soft music, candlelight and the works. Take one little piece, put it in your mouth, taste it, chew it, mix it with saliva and swirl it around your mouth. The more you enjoy life, the better things will work for you. The more you enjoy eating, the less it will cause problems for you. The purpose of the ritual is to experience the maximum amount of pleasure and satisfaction from eating. Have an abundance of food so you can eat until you are satisfied. If it takes two gallons of ice cream, do it! If you want to fast for two days afterwards, that is OK, too. The pleasure of the satisfaction makes it worthwhile.

Another good exercise is to take a deep breath between each bite. The purpose is to stay conscious and to notice how you hold your breath while eating. It is a question of getting oral satisfaction through breathing rather than "stuffing your tubes."

Remember, if you lose weight and gain beauty, then gaining is better than losing.

If you have been overweight or underweight for very long, you undoubtedly are already familiar with the literature on the subject. There are many processes that can be undertaken to recognize and deal with your ideas about food. The most positive of these have to do with learning to savor every bite you eat and giving yourself permission to experience the pleasure of eating. Doing these processes will increase your satisfaction not only with food but also with your life generally.

The following list of weight affirmations can be used as a starting point in reprogramming your mind to change your body. You will automatically think of others that perfectly suit your particular situation. Remember, losing weight and gaining beauty makes gaining better than losing!

WEIGHT AFFIRMATIONS

1. I like my body—and the more I like it, the more lovable it becomes.
2. My body automatically processes everything I eat to maintain my perfect weight of _____.
3. Everything I eat turns to health and beauty.
4. I deserve the pleasure that I am about to receive from eating.
5. I am losing weight and gaining beauty.
6. I am highly pleasing to myself whether I eat or not.
7. I am highly pleasing to my parents whether I eat or not.
8. The more I experience pleasure from eating, the more beautiful I become.
9. Food itself is not fattening; the instructions I give to the food control my results.
10. Infinite Intelligence within me always does the right thing to maintain my perfect weight of _____.
11. I now have enough time to enjoy eating while I am doing it.
12. That which is pleasurable no longer has any undesirable consequences.
13. The more satisfaction I experience, the less emptiness I experience.
14. My life and health are really sustained by the Light of God.
15. All food is good for me and I eat for pleasure.
16. My metabolism is responding to my new instructions.
17. I only eat when I fully enjoy it.
18. I have the right to change my parents rules about eating.
19. I deserve to be loved and I am OK whether I eat or not.

11 The Ten Commandments by Leonard Orr

The Ten Commandments are very useful when you understand what they mean. They are useful for maintaining bliss and peace, for producing abundance, for producing harmonious relationships, and for the satisfaction of using your own power. Practicing the Ten Commandments is the way to Heaven. Leonard suggests that people go back to church to free their minds. The easiest way to free yourself from your religious conditioning is to go back to the original environment (after you have been enlightened) and see how stultifying it was. Clean that stuff out so that you are really pure. Clean out the "stuff" that invalidates your personal divine power. ("The pure in heart shall see God.") Go back to your church and sit there until you are free of it. Then use your divine power to put life back into the churches and free your brothers and sisters from religious bondage.

Doing genuine spiritual work in your local church will expand your own growth. The Bible is an expression of eternal life. Since eternal life is always present in every point of space and time, then the Bible is only rightly interpreted when it reveals the truth of the present moment. Therefore, the Ten Commandments are not only ethical principles but, on the highest level, they are also declarations of spiritual reality.

Jesus condensed the Ten Commandments into two: First,

"Thou shalt love the Lord thy God with all thy heart, and with all thy soul, and with all thy mind, and with all thy strength." This is a summary of the first four Commandments. This Commandment says to love your God; to love God you must have a God. Where does God come from? The answer always ends up being in your mind. That is, the more accurately you describe your personal being, mind and body, the closer you get to self-mastery and to God. So your conception of yourself determines your conception of God. And the bigger your conception of yourself, the bigger your conception of God.

The second great Commandment summarizes the last six: "Thou shalt love thy neighbor as thy self." This Commandment makes other people equal to you. And it means that the quality of your self-esteem determines the value you have for other people. If you hate yourself, you'll hate other people; and if you hate others, it means you hate yourself. If there is a portion of yourself or a corner of your own mind of which you disapprove, you will disapprove of it when you see it in other people. (If you approve of your disapproval, however, it can lead to positive change.)

In order to understand the scriptures completely, *you* have to be a spiritual Master. And, if you are a spiritual Master, then you can write your own!

When you interpret the scriptures properly, as you have noticed with these Commandments, they are very simple: There is a *Presence* and there is a *Law*. The Presence is your own life (which is the space between your thoughts as well as during them). The Law is your own mind (which is your ability to think and the collections of your thoughts that have created your personal reality the way it is). The Law is that thought is creative. If you understand the following interpretation of the Ten Commandments, you are already a spiritual Master.

The Bible is the Book of Life which you write with your own mind. So the last judgment is every day. The day of judgment is any day that you notice what your reality is . . . or when you reap the results of the thoughts you have thought.

The Spiritual Interpretation of the Ten Commandments

I. Thou shalt have no other gods before me.

First you have to define *thou*. Thou is you. Then you have to define *me*. Me is you also. God is Thou and me (otherwise there is more than one God). Me is the God in everyone. God is the me in everyone. The me of you is the same as the me of me. The me of you and the me of me are one and the same—which is God. This Commandment says *I am God* or *You are God*. Since it is you who is God, then you have to create God. *Man created God in his own image.* (Humility = If you are God it is impossible to say anything too good about yourself). Me is the intuitive perception of your own being. Therefore, thou should not have other gods before the intuitive perception of your own being. The First Commandment produces spiritual enlightenment.

If there is only one God in the universe, then everything in the universe is part of God. This generates the doctrine of the Unity of Being and makes you God. However, God is bigger than your perceptions of God forever. (In the First Commandment we have the Presence.) When you are exalting or praising yourself, you are not invalidating God, because God is not outside of you. God is praised by your actions and your self-esteem. Knowing that you are God is the foundation of any healthy personality. It is not the end point of enlightenment; it is the beginning.

II. Thou shalt not bow down thyself unto any graven images.

How do you make a "graven image" of Infinite Being? It is impossible. You can particularize an idea into form, but when you make an idea into form, *you* are the creator. So to bow down to what you have created and worship it as your creator is ridiculous. If you acknowledge what you have created as your source, then you become limited by that source. To do that is to deny your own being, to invalidate and hate that being for its inability. And so, if you invalidate your own being, you will be self-punished. "I will visit the inequity of the third and fourth generations of them that hate me," which means that the results of the invalidations will persist as long as the invalidation. Or, in other words, the punishment of the sin will persist as long as people keep sinning. Obviously invalidating your own being will bring about confusion and misery.

In the Second Commandment we have the law, *thought is creative.* The law is the law of righteousness (right thinking) which is the Truth. The law of inequity (wrong thinking) is invalidating the Truth. This Commandment illustrates that the Ten Commandments are not just ethical principles which you are supposed to practice, but are laws of reality which you are practicing whether you like it or not.

All reality consists of images graven out of Infinite Being by thought. It is obviously ridiculous to think the created reality is the source, and to think so frustrates satisfaction and definitely limits progress.

III. Thou shalt not take the name of the Lord thy God in vain, for He will not hold him guiltless that taketh His Name in vain.

The name of the Lord is "I AM THAT I AM." So if you take "I AM THAT I AM" in vain, what happens? It means you use it without conscious intention. If you say "I AM sick" or "I AM poor" or "I am lonely" then you take the name of the Lord in vain if you don't desire poverty and illness. Whatever you put after I am, you become. You can demonstrate this oneness with telepathy, astral projection, etc.

Anytime you negate the intuitive perception of your own being, or any of the substantive qualities of being, like love and power, you will experience pain. And if you experience pain and have forgotten or don't understand how you created it, you won't have the strength to get rid of it. As soon as you acknowledge that you are creating the pain with your strength, then all you have to do is

invert the negative idea into the truth and the pain will disappear.
Affirmations are necessary when you are negating the truth.
Making an affirmation is a way of inverting or correcting your
negation, and after you have made the transformation, power and
bliss will flow into your consciousness.

There are basically two qualities of thought: Those thoughts
which are Being contemplating itself and its substantive qualities;
and Being contemplating a particular reality and making it take
form. Forms have a tendency to be eternal. You don't have to do
anything to keep the earth here. It will be here whether you worry
about it or not; and if you worry about it a whole lot, then you
won't be here and the earth will! The earth persists, and the
Biblical word for persistence is Everlasting.

As long as you honor and respect the name of the Lord
(yourself) then you create your own totally desirable reality.
Something undesirable, such as pain, is caused by negation of life.
A thought like "Nobody loves me" is invalidation of the truth.
Infinite Being is loving you every second, and between seconds,
and around seconds.

The name of the Lord is the revelation of the truth about life
which is both the Presence (of Infinite Being in your consciousness) and the Law of life (that thought is creative). Thought
creates. You create your universe according to the quality of your
thoughts. The first "I Am" is the quality of your thought.

IV. Remember the Sabbath to keep it holy.

The Fourth Commandent embodies the principles of rest, which
says it is time to stop working on your creation and relax; and so it
is the principle of completion. You work with an idea until it
manifests and, once it manifests, you don't have to work with it
anymore. The way that applies to the affirmations principle is that
when you work with an idea long enough, then you should leave it
alone and let it manifest. It is like a seed you plant—you don't dig
it up every day to see if it is growing! Once you have created something into form, leave it alone and enjoy it. Go on and build some-

thing else. When you operate from the standpoint of completed consciousness (the standpoint of rest), you have a lot more power than when you are working seven days a week. When you accept and understand that you have the right to rest anytime, things go well. Everyone has a cycle of work, however, and that cycle is whatever you determine it to be, six days, five days, whatever you want. We can judge intuitively what the cycle is. Something is complete when it fulfills your purpose.

Ultimately, everything is always at rest and everything is always completed. Incompletion has to be completed in order to be incompletion. If incompletion were not at rest or complete at the point of incompletion, then incompletion would not exist. In order for completion to exist, it has to be a complete incompletion. So everything is always in a state of completion and incompletion at the same time. Everything is at rest and at motion at the same time. The difference between rest and motion is ultimately your thought about it and continues only as long as you hold that thought. So the Fourth Commandment is a declaration of the truth that particular reality, or personal reality, is arbitrary. Every time you read this book, you will get something new out of it, which means you have never completed it. So every time your personal reality changes, this book will change. But if you read it once and get some value, then you have completed it.

The practical value of this is the certainty that you control your personality and therefore can always be at rest over it in your kingdom. So rest is the knowledge that there are no surprises except the ones you plan. Ultimate strength and ultimate power is rest. If you had absolute power, there would be nobody in the universe to resist you. If there is nothing to resist, then you don't have anything to do but rest. And so then you can create and destroy while at rest.

The first "day" of Genesis took place before the sun was created; how could you have a day, in the literal sense, when you don't have a sun? So a day can mean anything you want it to mean. The six days of creation symbolize whatever amount of time it takes you to manifest a particular reality or to reach a particular goal. Most people make the mistake of working longer than they should; they continue working on a goal after it has been completed. Therefore they never know they have completed it. The way you can realize that you've completed it is to rest from your effort and see if your reality self-destructs. This is the spirit of the Fourth Commandment.

A common example of our over-efforting can be seen in a relationship in which one continues trying to earn the other's love after already having it. If you do this then you never *experience* the other's love, you never experience the fact that you have a successful relationship. To keep doing things to earn the person's love invalidates that person's love. When the other expresses that invalidation, it makes you feel insecure and this will eventually destroy the relationship. You can never do enough to earn what you already have.

V. Honor thy father and thy mother that thy days may be long upon the land which the Lord thy God giveth thee.

To honor your father and mother means to honor the ideas they gave you, and to honor the ideas they gave you is to understand them. That means that if you understand the ideas and the thoughts that your parents gave you, then you will reject them or accept them based upon their quality and their contribution to your purposes. So, to honor your father and your mother is the whole idea of self-analysis. It combines the ideas of self-analysis and psychoanalysis—seeing how the ideas your father and mother gave you are creating your reality. And if you change your reality, then you will live in your consciousness as long as you desire.

The idea of physical immortality is assumed in all the Commandments. One of the verses Leonard likes from *The Upanishads* is, "Immortality is given to him who unravels the ignorance of his youth." This is a beautiful paraphrase of the Fifth Commandment.

Your father and mother are simply your past ideas. Your present reality is the child of your past ideas. In this Commandment, land is a symbol for consciousness. So "the Lord thy God" gives you your consciousness, which is the cosmos. Your created universe is your consciousness (which includes your life stream, your mind, your ability to think and chose thoughts, and also the realities you have created—from the stars to the chair you are sitting on). You have, at least, created your experience of it. And insofar as the stars enter your consciousness, you are the creator of those stars.

To practice this Commandment is to realize that there is no reality given to you by your family that is not subject to your personal choice. It is desirable to point out that most of your conditioning is positive and wonderful. But it takes very little negative thought or untruth to kill you, or to create enough misery to keep you from appreciating the beauty of life. It is obvious that if you think about all of life's beauties, you won't have time to think about anything else. Furthermore, if you love your body as much God loves your body, then it will last forever.

VI. *Thou shalt not kill.*

It is impossible to kill. From the standpoint of murderers and victims, you have to have victims in order to have murderers. So if the victim is a person who desires to be killed, then the murderer is victimized by the victim. The murderer is the servant of the victim. On a higher plane there is no such thing as death, because your physical body goes into the earth and it becomes fertilizer, fertilizer nourishes the apple tree and somebody comes along and eats the apples. The apples become a body and the cycle continues forever.

To kill means to deprive of existence something that wants to exist. If you are destroying something that wants to be destroyed, you are giving *life* to the desire to be destroyed. And you realize, ultimately, that the thing that is doing the killing is Infinite Being and Infinite Being is not killed and cannot be killed.

The superficial reality of this Commandment is that, if you destroy other people's bodies, then you are asking for your own body to be destroyed. The reason people kill other people is because of their own death urge. They are symbolically asking somebody to kill them. The Commandment means that to destroy human flesh will ultimately create the destruction of your own.

You can take this principle to its extreme. When you breathe, you inhale microorganisms that may get killed; if you are against killing to the extent that you stop breathing to save the microorganisms, then probably your existence won't be very meaningful. This Commandment has meaning only on an absolute level of the unity of Being: it is impossible for Spirit to destroy itself. The interpretation of this in regard to particular forms is totally arbitrary. When you eat plants and animals you are killing those forms.

Death is only possible in the sense that you can create or destroy particular forms. But you can't destroy your ability to re-create particular forms. So if you always have the ability to recreate your form, or other forms, then nothing is gone further than a thought away! To indulge in the thought that you can kill something keeps you from recreating it.

If you take the Commandment literally, then God is a murderer because He kills everybody. However, God really is not interested in destroying your physical body. If your physical body gets destroyed, it is your own fault. The idea that death is inevitable has killed more people than all other causes combined. This belief has no practical value if you are interested in the aliveness of your mind, spirit and body. The belief that death is inevitable is passing away like other universally held beliefs. (Example: that the world was flat and the center of the solar system.)

On the other hand, *believing* in physical immortality (or that death is NOT inevitable) can in no way harm you, if it is inevitable. If you are going to die anyway, caused by some force outside your control, it doesn't matter what you believe.

The practical value of the Commandment is to teach us not to indulge in a mortal mentality. There is a lot more to be said about this Commandment, but since you are God, you can figure it out yourself.

One other ultimate thing is if you could dematerialize and rematerialize your own body at will, would you call dematerializing it *killing?*

VII. Thou shalt not commit adultery.

The superficial definition of adultery is sleeping with a guy's wife or a woman's husband without their permission. Adultery really means the adulteration of your own thoughts. If you adulterate the First Commandment, then all you can do is commit adultery. As long as you honor yourself as God you are not adulterating the truth and then everything is OK. Because if you are God, you can decide that you are married today and that you are not married tonight (so you could sleep with another woman) and then you could decide you are married again tomorrow. If you are a woman, you can sleep with your husband last night, go out today and be a hooker and when you are through hooking, you can go back and be married again if you want to. If you are God, you have the right to do that. However, the other people are Gods also and when you mess around with other gods like this the consequences can be very heavy.

Adultery in human relations has to do with keeping agreements; and so, since you are the Pope, you have the power to give yourself absolution and the power to change agreements. Obviously, if you have the power to make agreements and you have the power to change agreements, you have total absolute power over your agreements. You can do anything you want with them. Things work out between two people however they decide it will work out. If they are two people who keep breaking agreements, then they are two people who keep their agreement to break their agreements.

In regard to sex, God makes love to everybody. Therefore, one person is as good as another. If a person has a spirit, a mind, and a body they are practicing the truth ultimately and all differences are ultimately a matter of personal opinion and taste. Of course, personal taste is OK.

It has always been our personal policy to not seduce or be seduced by individuals who are married or in heavy relationships. With us this policy is based upon respect for simplicity and their divine power.

VIII. Thou shalt not steal.

You are well aware by now that by the use of affirmations, by improving the quality of your thoughts, and by having a prosperity consciousness, you will acquire anything you need or want. Stealing is primarily motivated by the need to acquire something not otherwise obtainable. Since you now have all the means of acquision you will ever need, there is no need to steal. If you take another person's possessions, you are invalidating that you are Infinite Being. So, therefore, stealing comes from breaking the First Commandment.

To take another person's possession or steal from them is to steal from yourself (i.e. if you are stealing from your own power, your own authority, your own happiness, and your own Divine Identity) then don't be surprised if people take your possessions to symbolize what you are doing to yourself. So if you are stealing from yourself, don't be surprised if other people help you and rip you off.

If a person did take a possession of yours and you were not stealing from yourself, then you would consider it to be a gift and it would come back to you multiplied. The thief would be activating the spending law for you!

IX. Thou shalt not bear false witness.

The Bible implies that God cannot lie because everything He says becomes true. By applying the First Commandment, the same is true of you. You cannot lie because everything you say is true, as long as you believe it to be true and desire to manifest it. And so there is no such thing as false witness. So if you say something to one person about another and if the person you say it to believes you, then it is true for that person and he creates it for himself. But even though it is true for him it may not be true for the person you told it about. If it is not true about the person you told it about, then there is no lie there . . . so where is the lie? The only lie is in believing there is a lie, that there can be such a thing as a lie. The person who believes the lie has to live with it, not the person it was told about.

The way Leonard applies this practically is to not believe anything anyone tells him unless it is for the highest good of himself and everyone concerned.

X. Thou shalt not covet thy neighbor's house, possessions, wives, etc.

The interpretation of this Commandment is similar to that of the Eighth Commandment. To covet anything your neighbor has is to deny your power to manifest it for yourself. To covet is based upon the feeling that you don't have the right to something or the power to get something yourself. If you covet your neighbor's boat, then you are affirming you don't have the power to get one yourself, which makes it harder, if not impossible, for you to get your own.

To covet is to believe that your neighbor will not give you permission to use his possession. To believe that your neighbor will not give you permission is to believe that he is not you, which is a denial of the First Commandment. If you deny that he is not you, the he obviously won't give you permission.

On the other hand, to take other people's possessions without their permission is to expose yourself to the power of their divine wrath.

Therefore, practicing this Commandment maintains a simple and happy life.

Epilogue
by Sondra

Writing this book was such a powerful emotional experience that I sometimes got sick—other times I put my head down on the typewriter and cried. Once, the typewriter "went mad" and got stuck on automatic carriage return and started going "Zoom-zoom-zoom" hysterically. I thought it was going to blow up! I went through a kind of rebirth cycle during the typing of one draft of the rebirth chapter. I re-lived the trauma done to my spine coming out of the birth canal and ended up having to go to a body manipulation therapist to get my spine back in place. I can now breathe better than ever before.

For a period of five days while writing the Immortality chapter the joints of my fingers became very painful and I developed psuedo-arthritis. This put me in a panic and I ran to Leonard, absolutely terrified that I would never be able to type again. (At that time I was also experiencing aching in the bones, loss of hearing and crusting and scaling of the skin.) He said "Oh, this is great! You are feeling safe enough now to experience your old age early and it means you won't have to go through it later." He was so pleased that I actually left his room feeling elated about being senile at thirty-five, and even more intrigued about the effects of choosing immortality.

Once I got up very early to type in the dining room of Tom and Val's house in Walton, New York. You can imagine my shock when I went to my typing area and found the entire manuscript strewn all over the floor. Since the pages were not yet numbered I really went crazy. When Gary saw that the pages were chewed on some corners, he informed me of the culprit: the cat! We never did find one page.

It was incredible fun, anyway, and the places in which we wrote it are worth mentioning. The chapter on politics Leonard spontaneously dictated to me inside the Haleakala Crater, Maui, Hawaii, on the Bicentennial Fourth of July. I wrote it frantically on some yellow paper I had stuffed into my back pack. When he finished I asked him if he realized what date it was; neither of us had planned it, but I got very excited when I saw the historical implication. We reviewed much of the book in the middle of the night aboard planes, buses and trains in Europe or India. That seemed to be the best time for me to capture Leonard, who is always in great demand. Sometimes in India I would get him up at 6:30, and while he was still half asleep, I would coax out of him his latest comments. Another good place to catch him, as always, was while he was in the bathroom. Once I was rebirthing him and he got very inspired. He jumped up in the middle of the rebirth and started pacing the floor. I was without my pad, so I grabbed some hotel stationery. Consequently, at the end of our trip I wound up with stuff written on hotel stationery, napkins and menus. There was no place to make copies, so I usually slept with this manuscript.

Once we took a very long drive in Leonard's silver Mazda. We played Beethoven, Chopin, and Mendelssohn and I read what we had done so far. When I came to the part about my first rebirth and my breathing release, I totally relived the joy of that moment and burst into tears. Leonard reached into the back window well for some tissues and lovingly told me to take my time. He was just as tuned in to that memory as I was and I felt my tears of relief for both of us. As I was reading over the chapter on rebirthing, Leonard's ankles began to pain him. So he stuck his right foot in my lap so that I could massage it, and put his left foot on the gas—then he returned his right foot to the gas and crossed over his left foot to me. It was pretty funny to watch him drive like that. (He was recalling the pain at birth of being held upside down by his ankles.) I wasn't able to be in the driver's seat while discussing the manuscript. I tried it. Describing to my friend Jackie how it felt to write this book and how my typewriter went berserk, I drove slightly off the road and had a blowout. So as you can see, I have been very emotionally involved in this book and it was a fabulous enlightenment process for me. You might say I really lived it! The book was actually finished at Mt. Shasta. This was unplanned (by me, anyway). Gary and I were driving along late one night and became inspired to add one more part. We were delighted to complete the book at the Mystical Shrine of the Ascended Masters.

Appendices

Appendix A

A Completion Checklist For Rebirthees and Rebirthers
by Leonard Orr
301 Lyon Street
San Francisco, California 94117
(415) 929-1743

STEP 1: Do ten to twenty relaxed intuitive connected rhythmical breathing sessions with a trained rebirther. That is, at least ten ordinary "dry" rebirthing sessions. With most people the dramatic emotional and physical drama stops within ten sessions, and they are able to maintain the connected breathing rhythm without drama for one hour. With regular practice of the breathing rhythm over a long period, rebirthing produces less and less eventful sessions. Breath mastery produces the experience of the body as an energy system that can be healthy and calm, blissful state of mind becomes ordinary. After ten to twenty sessions, the accumulated tension of a lifetime gets dissolved and daily practice maintains a wonderful state of spiritual purification with a sense of mental and physical cleanliness that gets taken for granted probably too soon and too easily. Going for the drama and "acting out" instead of going for the release through breathing can make this level of clarity take dozens or hundreds of sessions to get to the same point. Relaxed, intuitive breathing rhythm is the key.

STEP 2: Making your overall transformation easy on you and everyone else. (a) By the tenth session you should have thoroughly exposed yourself to the philosophy of physical immortality, the psychology of unraveling the personal death urge, and some basic principles of body mastery. (b) You should have developed the habit of attending seminars regularly to widen your perspective on rebirthing and related self-improvement topics. (c) You should know what support spiritual family and community means. (d) You should have plenty of experience practicing with affirmations. (e) You should be familiar with the spiritual purification exercises list, with Excellence in Rebirthing statement, and with rebirthing organizations like Rebirth International.

STEP 3: After ten sessions, you should trade sessions with your rebirther in case you happen to be spiritually, intellectually or psychologically more advanced than your rebirther. Since you're trading sessions, this also makes the rest of your rebirthing process free. Good rebirthers deserve to be paid for the first ten sessions. Rebirthers currently charge from $1 to $100 per session. I recommend that you trade at least three sessions with your rebirther before you break your rebirthing relationship. Then you can start rebirthing, which should start by trading sessions with other rebirthees.

STEP 4: After ten sessions or as soon as dramatic psychological or emotional drama stops, which may be before or after ten sessions, you should start rebirthing yourself. You should continue rebirthing yourself until you can maintain a relaxed connected intuitive breathing rhythm for at least an hour. At this point, you should also practice doing twenty connected breaths whenever you feel like it, especially when you are uptight or angry or experiencing other physical or emotional drama.

STEP 5: After you have completed ten sessions and sometimes before, if you get stuck, or if you have what might be termed an angry or hostile personality, you should do your rebirthing sessions with a pen, pencil or toothbrush handle between your teeth. This bit between your teeth technique permits spirit to dissolve your anger. This also will cure you from grinding your teeth during sleep, which is bad on teeth as well as rest. Anger is defined as misdirected energy. If you experience anger often, I recommend that you use it for accomplishment instead of destruction, which may be your own and ultimately will be your own.

STEP 6: Anytime after ten dry breathing sessions when you feel like it you should start wet rebirthing. A pretty complete guide on warm water rebirthings is included in the book, "Rebirthing in the New Age." Basically you should maintain the breathing rhythm that you've mastered both in warm water or cold until you no longer have any emotional or physical drama. It is recommended that you do your first sessions with a trained rebirther in a hot tub until you feel comfortable doing them alone.

STEP 7: The basic cold water rebirthing technique is to get into the connected breathing rhythm. While maintaining a connected rhythm, put one inch of one foot into the cold water. When your foot becomes comfortable, move in an inch at a time until your whole body is submerged. If at any time you lost the breathing rhythm, you should stop, back out and start over again. Some people take weeks of practice before they are masters of cold water rebirthing. You may want to wear a jacket or other clothing on the top half of your body while you're working on the lower half. The object is not discomfort or pain, but rather increasing the margins of comfort and pleasure. Rebirthing is the New Yoga of comfort and pleasure. If God had wanted you to be cold, he would have formed you in an ice cube instead of a warm womb. Warm and cold water rebirthing releases basic temperature trauma and makes your physical body more pleasurable all the time.

STEP 8: Spiritual Healing: The breath of life as mentioned in Genesis is the source of every person's breath and is the source of all healing. If you stop breathing, you will get very, very sick. So sick, in fact, that your body will return to the dust and you will prove the Bible right. The body is created out of the breath by the mind.

Therefore, the breath is the source of the body and simple breathing and upgrading the quality of your thoughts about your body can heal everything. The touch of loving massage will obviously accelerate the healing process. The truth is there are no illnesses, only healings. What is called sickness is only a healing in progress. All illnesses and accidents are either the spirit and body attempting to heal the mind or the spirit and mind attempting to heal the body. All negative symptoms are ultimately created by negative thought, but occasionally, an obsolete positive thought that is overdue for a transformation. If your healing is not proceeding as efficiently as it could be, it is because you are not breathing enough or not thinking enough. It is obviously necessary to give up your negative belief system about your symptoms even if they have been given to you by an authority that you respect. Common sense leads us to the conclusion that we ourselves have had the most training in living in our body and mind and are therefore the best authority for them. We are all physicians who must heal ourselves.

More details on these levels of completion will be added in another chapter. It is recommended that you complete your own breath mastery, that you become a competent rebirther, that you learn how to train rebirthers, and if you so desire, go on to train rebirther trainers. If every breather shares breath mastery with at least ten to one hundred other people, it won't take long for everybody in the world to enjoy the benefits of breath mastery.

Appendix B:

Suggested Books and Tapes

The following books and tapes contain some of the most valuable ideas to be found anywhere. I encourage you to use these products to further your growth and success. Reading and listening is a wonderful and effective way to use the suggestion principle. Take charge of your life. Deliberately build the consciousness you want now by reading and listening to these and other positive products. Surround yourself with good ideas.

I suggest that you pick one or more of these books and tapes that appeal to you and use it to expand your success. Get into the habit of self-improvement. A positive and enlightened consciousness is your most valuable possession.

Suggested Reading

Books by Sondra Ray

The Celebration of Breath
Sondra Ray

$7.95, paper, 204 pages
Celestial Arts, Berkeley, CA
This is the latest book on Rebirthing, sharing new advancements in
Rebirthing, Breath Awareness and Healing.

Loving Relationships
Sondra Ray

$6.95, paper, 176 pages
Celestial Arts, Berkeley, CA
Gain deep insights into your relationships with your lover, parents,
children, boss, friends and your relationship with yourself. Find out
why your relationships turn out the way the do, and improve the
quality of all your relationships.

CONTENTS INCLUDE: Part One: THE SECRETS. God. Get Enlightened. Use Affirmations. Get Rebirthed. Handle Your Unconscious Death Urge. Love Yourself. Love Your Body. Clear Up The Ten Patterns. Handle Old Relationships. The Highest Spiritual Thought. Purpose of Relationship. Surrender. Part Two: MORE ABOUT RELATIONSHIPS. Werner Erhard. Loving Relationships Training. Personal Accounts from the L.R.T. Part Three: RELATIONSHIPS WITH IMMORTALISTS. Bobby. Fred. Jim. Bob. Bill. The Making of A Trainer.

Those of you who have taken the Loving Relationships Training will immediately recognize these chapter headings. Much of the book is directly from the information in the training, which Sondra has been developing and perfecting for years.

As with *I Deserve Love,* the book is very clearly and simply written, and designed for immediate and successful personal use.

I Deserve Love
Sondra Ray

$6.95, paper, 128 pages
Celestial Arts, Berkeley, CA
Love, sex, and relationships. Using affirmations to have what you want, and to expand your self-esteem. Affirmations are "positive thoughts you hold in mind to produce desired results." Why and how affirmations work is the powerful topic of this book. Through writing and stating affirmations, thought patterns become progressively more positive. You then tune in to the "universal consciousness," attracting those on higher and higher vibration levels. Affirmations such as "I deserve love," and "I deserve sexual pleasure," are shown to work in a matter of days. This is strikingly illustrated by the various case studies which Sondra presents throughout the book. The book is filled with positive ideas on sex, love, relationships and self esteem.

The Only Diet There Is
Sondra Ray

$6.95, paper, 156 pages
Celestial Arts, Berkeley, CA
"Driving up the California coast one glorious winter day, Sondra Ray read me the text of this book. It was stunning. The message was so simple, so true, I was amazed it hadn't been written before. As often with Sondra's ideas, I volunteered to be the first 'subject,' the first tried-and-tested 'experiment.' Would this really work? The next day I began this unusual diet. Life has never been quite the same. By the end of the week, I'd lost several pounds but, more important, I was so in love with life and myself I had the self-worth to create a beautiful body. Within one month I had lost fifteen pounds, achieving my perfect body weight. The theory is simple. Though we might think it is our negative eating habits that have kept us unattractive and unhealthy, it is really our negative thoughts and feelings."
From the Preface by Linda Thistle, Ph.D.
This book is about much more than weight and dieting. It is about improving your relationship with your self and your body.

The Truth About Psychology

From Here to Greater Happiness
Joel and Champion Teutsch

$2.95, paper, 176 pages
Price/Stern/Sloan, Los Angeles, CA
A clear and simple explanation of how the mind works. Examples of personal laws in action.

The Creative Process in the Individual
Thomas Troward

$7.95, cloth
Dodd, Mead & Co., N.Y., NY
This is an excellent book on metaphysics — how life works. Other books by the same author are good, too. (Dore' Lectures; Edinburgh Lectures; Bible Mystery & Bible Meaning)

Your Inner Child of the Past
Hugh Missildine

$2.95, paper
Simon and Schuster, N.Y., NY
This is a clear, loving psychological book about childhood. It gives case histories which you can use to locate you own childhood patterns.

Spiritual Psychology
Jim Morningstar, Ph.D.

$8.00, paper, 180 pages
Spiritual Psychology Press, Milwaukee, WI
A brilliant synthesis of Contemporary Psychology, Holistic Health, and Modern Metaphysics. An integration of the body, mind, and spirit for the new age.

Rebirthing

Rebirthing in the New Age
Leonard Orr and Sondra Ray

$9.95, paper, 320 pages
Celestial Arts, Berkeley, CA
This is the original book on Rebirthing. It is considered a necessary textbook for those interested in Rebirthing.

Rebirthing: The Science of Enjoying All Your Life
Phil Laut

$7.95, paper
Trinity Publications, San Rafael, CA
This book describes how rebirthing works in a simple and detailed way. Contents include: The truth about being human; Rebirthing; How to create your reality; Your past and you; Immortalist philosophy; Your future and you.

Birth Without Violence
Dr. Frederic Leboyer

$11.95, cloth, 128 pages
Random House, Westminister, MD
Birth from the baby's viewpoint. Reading this book can help you remember your own birth and the first (nonverbal) conclusions you made about life. Beautifully written and illustrated with photographs of blissful and aware babies. This book is requried reading for the Rebirthing process. It is also an excellent book for anyone who is planning on being involved in the birth of a child. Rediscover the divine child within you.

Secret Life of the Unborn Child
Dr. Thomas Verny, M.D.

$6.95, paper
Summit Books, N.Y., NY
Synthesizing for the first time the latest findings from all scientific disciplines dealing with the unborn, including Dr. Verny's pioneering work in prenatal psychology. *The Secret Life of the Unborn Child* demonstrates that from the sixth month of intrauterine life (and sometimes even earlier) the unborn child is a feeling, experiencing, remembering being who responds to and is deeply influenced by his environment.

Money and Prosperity

Money Is My Friend
Phil Laut

$5.00, paper
Trinity publications, San Rafael, CA
"One of the best books available about prosperity consciousness."
The author probes every area of life that could be blocking the reader
from reaching his full potential. This book covers the topic of
"money in abundance" in depth.

Moneylove
Jerry Gillies

$2.95, paper
Warner Books, New York, NY
Particularly good for freeing up your attitudes about money.

The Richest Man in Babylon
George Clason

$2.95, paper, 160 pages
Bantam Books, New York, NY
A wonderful primer on the 4 laws of wealth. Recommended at
money seminars as the best basic book about money. Written in par-
ables. "A lean purse is easier to cure than to endure."

Physical Immortality
Leonard Orr

$9.95, paper, 80 pages
Celestial Arts, Berkeley, CA
In depth discussion of immortalist philosophy. An account of the immortal master Herakahn Baba in India. Socological implications of
physical immortality.

The Door of Everything
by Ruby Nelson

$3.95, paper, 180 pages
DeVorss & Co., Marina del Rey, CA
A wonderful statement of Immortalist Philosophy.

The Immortalist
Alan Harrington

$5.95, paper, 316 pages
Celestial Arts, Berkeley, CA
An alternative to the belief systems that accept and educate people for inevitable death. It proposes that "the time has come for man to get rid of the intimidating gods in his own head, to grow up out of his cosmic inferiority complex, to bring his disguised desire for eternal life into the open and go after what he really wants — the only state he will settle for — divinity." "Mr. Harrington may have written the most important book of our time." —Gore Vidal

Beyond Mortal Boundaries
Annalee Skarin

$4.95, paper, 356 pages
DeVorss & Co., Marina Del Rey, CA
Analee Skarin recognized the message of life eternal — physical immortality — through study of the Bible. Her book is an extremely power affirmation of life and the unlimited power of God through and in any person.

The Life and Teachings Of The Masters Of The Far East
Baird Spalding

$4.00 per volume, 5 volumes, paper
DeVorss & Co., Marina Del Rey, CA
An account of American scientists who visited and lived with immortal masters in the Himalayas around the turn of the century. From the introduction:

"During our stay — 3½ years — we contacted the great masters of the Himilayas... They permitted us to enter into their lives intimately, and we were thus able to see the actual workings of the Great law as demonstrated by them... They supply everything needed for their daily wants directly from the universe, including food, clothing, and money. They have so far overcome death that many of them now living are over 500 years old...." Full of uplifting ideas. They explain how they do it and how you can do the same.

Psychological Immortality
Jerry Gillies

$12.95, cloth, 256 pages
Richard Marek, New York, NY
A synthesis of science and immortalist philosophy. Exercises to expand aliveness.

Hariakhan Baba: Known, Unknown
Hari Dass

$2.50, paper
Sri Rama Foundation, Davis, CA
Hariakhan Baba is an immortal master of India. He has appeared for thousands of years throughout the Himalayan districts. This book contains stories, interviews and photographs never before published in the West; 18 photographs.

Suggested Listening

Spiritual Psychology

As A Man Thinketh
Leonard Orr

$12.00
Approximately one hour cassette
Produced by Life Unlimited (see address below)
Recorded positive version of James Allen's classic essay on the power of thought in all areas of life. Designed for repeated listening. Use this tape as a tool for self-analysis and as an affirmation.
Also available: AS A WOMAN THINKETH is the same essay with a woman's voice and pronouns. (also $12.00)

Rebirthing

Recreating Your Ideal Birth
Rima Beth Star and Glen Smyly

$15.00
30 Minutes each side.
Produced by Life Unlimited (see address below)
This is a cassette tape of a guided visualization process with a music background. It starts with relaxation, leading you back in time prior to conception. You then picture your conception, growth in the womb, birth and post birth experiences in the way you would like them to have been. Side Two is filled with affirmations on forgiveness and healing of your birth experience.

The Rebirth Seminar
Leonard Orr

$18.00   2 One hour cassette tapes (Live)
Produced by Life Unlimited (see address below)
The complete rebirth seminar, given in February 1977 by Leonard Orr, inventor of rebirthing and founder of Theta Seminars. Includes: What rebirthing is. The purpose and results of being rebirthed. How rebirthing was invented. What to expect in being rebirthed. Suggested follow up. Life energy and breathing. The breathing release. Healing, health and rebirthing. How rebirthing works. A model of the mind. The Rebirth seminar is a recommended prerequisite for being rebirthed. The tape is valuable whether or not you plan to be rebirthed.

Birth Separation
Barrie Konicov

$10.00
This is a cassette tape 45 minutes on a side.
The titles available on side two of the tape are GOOD HEALTH or PARENTAL DISAPPROVAL. The birth experience for most people is very traumatic. It can be the source of many physical ailments. This tape will help correct your breathing and release the negative feelings of your past that surround your birth. This hypnotic tape is designed for repeated use.

Good Health
Barrie Konicov

$10.00
Cassette tape, 45 minutes on a side.
This is a guided visualization hypnotic tape designed to improve your health. Those that have used it report amazing changes in their health, both mentally and physically. There are many titles available on side two. The most popular are BIRTH SEPARATION and TELL YOUR FEELINGS HOW TO FEEL.

Money and Prosperity

Money Seminar
Leonard Orr

$30.00
Produced by Life Unlimited (see address below)
4 tape set, Over 4 hours (Recorded Live)
These ideas have doubled and tripled the incomes of hundreds of people. The tapes include: The four laws of wealth. The most valuable idea in the universe. The relationship between money and love. What a prosperity consciousness is, and how to develop it. How to increase your income while doing what you enjoy most. Practical tools to have and enjoy any level of prosperity you desire. Dealing with bills. Spending. The savings principle. Keys to investing in stocks and real estate. The best investment there is. Prosperity affirmations. Financial independence — what it is and how to achieve it. How to end taxes. This tape may be used repetitively as a tool in mastering prosperity consciousness. It will pay for itself.

Money and the Five Biggies
Leonard Orr

$18.00
Two one-hour cassettes
Produced by Life Unlimited (see address below)
Leonard's classic money seminar, recorded live at the Rolf Institute. Includes using your mind to produce prosperity, the five basic blocks to wealth, and how to attain success consciousness. Plus valuable hints on budgeting, spending, saving, investing and prospering.

Live Long and Prosper
Jerry Gillies

$59.95, 12 Part Album
A 12 part course in abundance and success on 6 cassettes featuring Jerry Gillies, with all-new material inspired by his bestselling books,

MONEYLOVE and PSYCHOLOGICAL IMMORTALITY. Includes: A SENSE OF PURPOSE; THE SUCCESS HABIT; THE CREATIVE SELF; DECISION/COMMITMENT: FINANCIAL SELF CONFIDENCE; TAKE YOUR TIME; VISUALIZING SUCCESS, and a report packed with ideas for CREATIVE CASSETTE LISTENING. These tapes really work!

Your Ideal Relationship With Money
Sondra Ray

$10.00   Approximately 30 Minutes/side Cassette Tape.
Produced by Life Unlimited (see address below)
Fill your mind with prosperity the easy way with this beautiful affirmations tape. The tape contains Sondra's highest and best ideas about prosperity and money in affirmation form. Repetitive listening (with an open mind) will free you from all financial limitation by bringing up and dissolving any ideas in conflict with the positive ideas presented. The masterful musical background by Raphael makes listening a pleasure and helps to slide the ideas right into your subconscious. This is a wonderful way to practice the prosperity ideas presented in some of our other products. Both sides are identical.

Prosperity Plus
Rev. Ike

$12.00
Full of positive ideas about money. Contains an excellent success and prosperity visualization.

Money Prosperity
Barrie Konicov

$10.00
This is a cassette tape with a day version on one side and a night version on the other. This tape has a relaxation process and a guided visualization on overcoming barriers to success and a series of posi-

tive affirmations. It is designed for daily use to build a prosperity consciousness. Begin preparing your consciousness to attract the riches you deserve today!

Physical Immortality

Unravelling The Birth/Death Cycle
by Leonard Orr

$18.00 2 tape set, approximately 2 hours (Live)
Produced by Life Unlimited (see address below)
An excellent tape on 2 of the 5 Biggies: Birth and Death. Why do people die? There is an unconscious link between the patterns set up at birth and the time and circumstances of your death. Death is not inevitable. This powerful tape explores the possibility of unravelling your own programming toward death. You will experience greater aliveness now as you reclaim control over the destiny of your physical body. Depression, failure and hopelessness will become things of the past. Explore youthing as an alternative to aging. Family patterns. The unconscious death urge and how it operates. Affirmations. One of Leonard's best.

Spiritual Purification
Leonard Orr

$18.00   Two cassette tapes (Live), Approximately 3 hours.
Produced by Life Unlimited (see address below)
Specific practical techniques for purifying your body and mind. The benefits and necessity of spiritual purification are discussed. Many of these methods are collected from Leonard's visits with Immortal Masters in India. This is the tape for developing practical mastery over your physical body — the practical side of physical immortality.

Affirmations

Your Ideal Loving Relationship
Sondra Ray/Raphael

$10.00
Approximately 45 Minutes/side Cassette Tape
Produced by Life Unlimited (see address below)
Here is the perfect companion to Sondra's book. Just lie back, relax, switch on the tape player, and listen to incredibly beautiful music accompanied by the highest available positive thoughts on Loving Relationships. This is an affirmations tape, intended for repeated listening. Sondra suggests playing it while lying down, bathing, driving, or anytime you can relax and let it slide into your subconscious. The music was created by Raphael specifically for these affirmations. Those of you who have heard him perform know that he has the ability to capture the exact vibration of an idea, and transmit it through music. Each of his compositions with Sondra uniquely fit the meaning of the affirmations, and blend perfectly into an irresistible harmonious whole. The affirmations cover a full range of relationship ideas — attracting and keeping your perfect partner, fulfillment and depth in the relationship, successful communication, harmony, and support, getting exactly what you want, resolving old patterns, and more. Both sides are identical.

Your Ideal Relationship With Sex
Sondra Ray

$10.00
Approximately 24 Minutes/side Cassette Tape
Produced by Life Unlimited (see address below)
Sexual Pleasure is your divine birthright. This tape is designed by Sondra to free your mind of limiting beliefs about sex, such as guilt, fear, inhibition, etc. Through the use of affirmations, results you can expect include the ability to relax and be yourself freely in sex, freedom to honor your own desires and standards regarding sex. Clarity about your purpose in sex, increased intensity and duration of sexual

pleasure, being more comfortable with your sexuality and sensuality and certainty that pleasure, and sex, are good, and divinely approved. Raphael has created a sensual musical background especially for these affirmations. Both sides are identical.

Your Ideal Relationship With Your Body And Weight
Sondra Ray

$10.00
Approximately 24 Minutes/side Cassette Tape
Produced by Life Unlimited (see address below)
This affirmation tape trains your mind to have power over your body and what your body does with the food you eat. You establish the goal of your perfect weight and use those affirmations to bring it into being. You will also learn to love, or expand your love, for your body. The tape includes a specially composed musical background by Raphael. Both sides are identical.

How to Obtain These Books and Tapes

The prices listed above are accurate at the time of this printing, and may change. Many of the books are available in bookstores. To make it easy for you, I have arranged with LIFE UNLIMITED to carry all of the products listed above.

Write or call for a free catalog:
LIFE UNLIMITED
8125 Sunset Ave., Suite 204E
Fair Oaks, CA 95628
(916) 967-8442

To order the products listed above:

1. List the titles you want,
2. Include your name and shipping address,
3. Add $1.75 for shipping and handling plus .35¢ per title.
4. California residents add sales tax.
5. Make your check or money order to
    LIFE UNLIMITED.
    (Checks must be drawn on a U.S. bank.)

Or call and charge it (Visa or Mastercard). There is a 4% handling fee on telephone orders.

Readers interested in obtaining information on Rebirthing or LRT should write the following addresses:

For information concerning LRT and Sondra Ray

LRT
145 West 87th Street
New York, NY 10024
(212) 799-7323 — 7324

For information concerning Rebirthing in your area call:

Rebirth International
(1-800-641-4645) ext. 232

LRT INTERNATIONAL
145 WEST 87th STREET
NEW YORK, NY 10024
(212) 799-7324

NEW YORK
Meg Kane
34 West 85th St., Apt 1
New York, N.Y. 10024
(212) 580-8031

Judy Roberts
114 West 76th St., Apt BR
New York, N.Y. 10023
(212) 362-0083

BOSTON
Jose and Nice Santiago
P.O. Box 2627
Cambridge, MA 02238
(617) 864-0373

ATLANTA
Jim and Pru Collier
202 Ansley Villa Drive
Atlanta, GA 30324
(404) 872-9570

FLORIDA
Mikela Green
2600 Emerald Way North
Deerfield, FL 33442
(305) 428-4940

SAN FRANCISCO
Ken and Maureen Richards
1430 43rd Avenue
San Francisco, CA 94122
(415) 759-7575

SEATTLE
David & Doreen Tannenbaum
P.O. Box 22704
Seattle, WA 98122
(206) 236-0228

DENVER
Kate Lessley
2071 Grape Street
Denver, CO 80207
(303) 321-2735

LOS ANGELES
Rhonda Levand
1251 Fairburn Ave.
Los Angeles, CA 90024
(213) 470-4501

Manny Stamatakis
3406 Glendon Ave., #8
Los Angeles, CA 90034
(213) 202-0499

LONDON
Gillian Steel
Colne Denton
Old Ferry Wharf
Cheyne Walk
London SW10 England
011-441-352-3977

Diana Roberts
9D Claverton Street
London SW1V 3AY England
01-630-1501

AUSTRALIA
Melbourne:
Yvonne and Vincent Betar
44 Rae Street
Fitzroy North, Victoria 3068
61-3-481-5302

Sydney:
Wayne & Katrina O'Donovan
9-96 Ourimbah Road
Mosmin 2088
New South Wales
02-908-3848

ISRAEL
Ron and Miri Gilad
Hashahaf 21
Hofit 40295
053-96121
and in the U.S.:
Gilad
342 West 85th St., #18
New York, N.Y. 10024
(212) 595-1369

Sondra's tape
YOUR IDEAL RELATIONSHIP WITH YOUR BODY AND WEIGHT

Affirmations for losing weight with music in the background.

Send $12.50 (includes tax and postage) to:

Life Unlimited
8125 Sunset, 204-O
Fair Oaks, CA 95628
(916) 967-8442

Write for a free catalog of tapes, related books, and other products available.